STONEWELL
HEALING PRESS

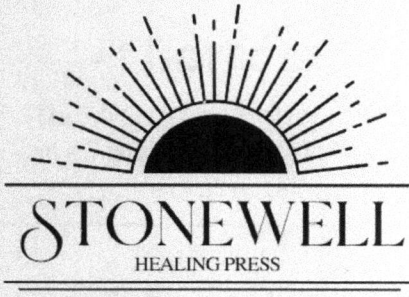

Thank you for being here. We're honored to walk beside you.

M. Tourangeau
Stonewell Healing Press

TABLE OF CONTENTS

SECTION 1 -   12

When Loss Hits Early –
Navigating the Shock of
Miscarriage

SECTION 2-   38

Grieving the Unseen –
Acknowledging the Loss That
Can't Be Held

SECTION 3 -   62

The Weight of Silence –
Navigating Expectations
and Conversations After
Loss

SECTION 4 -   84

Blaming My Body – Shame,
Guilt, and the Physicality of
Loss

SECTION 5-   104

Other People's Reactions –
When the World Doesn't Get
It

SECTION 6   130

Pregnancy After Loss – Hope,
Fear, and Not Trusting the Joy
Yet

Stonewell Healing Press

TABLE OF CONTENTS

SECTION 7 -   **148**

Already a Parent – Making Space for Grief When You Have to Keep Going

SECTION 8-   **168**

When Family Doesn't Understand – Dealing with Dismissive, Hurtful, or Silent Reactions

SECTION 9 -   **190**

The World Moves On – But I'm Still Not Okay

SECTION 10 -   **210**

Shadows and Shame – When Grief Feels Like Failure

SECTION 11 -   **228**

Letting Go Doesn't Mean Forgetting

BONUS SECTION   **250**

Redefining the Future – Holding Hope After Loss

Stonewell Healing Press

Dedicated to those who had to bury
a piece of their heart.

STONEWELL HEALING PRESS

HOW TO USE THIS WORKBOOK

Take your time with this. The more you pause to really think about each question and answer honestly, the more space you create for reflection. And with deeper reflection, this experience can open up new understanding and healing you might not expect.

Be honest with yourself—there's no judgment here. This is your private space. If you want, you can even throw this book away or burn it later to keep your secrets safe. That said, be mindful of how much you dive in. Healing and reflection around tough, sensitive topics can bring up strong feelings—and yes, it can get triggering. So here's your gentle trigger warning.

The real progress comes when you practice the skills, not just read about them. The more you try them out in your life, the more helpful this workbook will be.

ASSESSMENT

WHERE AM I NOW?

Before we begin, take a moment to honestly check in with yourself by rating these statements on a scale from 1 (not at all) to 10 (completely):

1-10

1. I feel able to acknowledge and sit with my grief without judgment.

2. I feel compassion for myself when I experience shame, guilt, or self-blame.

3. I feel able to talk about my miscarriage with others in a way that feels safe and supported.

4. I am able to hold my love for the baby I lost while also engaging in my daily life.

5. I feel capable of imagining a future that includes hope, joy, or possibility.

6. I feel I can honor my grief through rituals, memory practices, or reflective exercises.

7. I am able to notice and regulate my emotional and bodily responses when grief arises.

8. I feel empowered to define my healing process on my own terms, without pressure from others.

SECTION ONE

When Loss Hits Early – Navigating the Shock of Miscarriage

When you first experience a miscarriage, the grief can feel like an overwhelming wave — a deep, hollow sensation that strikes unexpectedly. You might have been planning, dreaming, or even just beginning to get excited, and in an instant, everything changes. The shock can be paralyzing. It might feel like you're suspended in time, unable to fully grasp the magnitude of what's happening, yet deeply aware of the loss.

This section is here to sit with you in that moment of confusion and disorientation. Grief is often not a linear path, and the shock of miscarriage can leave you feeling numb, disbelieving, or even distant from your own emotions. It's okay to feel like your world has suddenly tilted, as though you're struggling to find your footing. The purpose here is not to rush through the pain but to give yourself permission to feel what you need to feel, without judgment. It's natural to wonder if you'll ever feel "normal" again, or if the weight of this loss will always haunt you. What's important is to recognize that your body, mind, and heart are beginning a process of deep healing — even if it doesn't feel like it right now. In this section, we'll explore how shock can manifest in both your body and mind, and begin to create a space where healing can slowly take root.

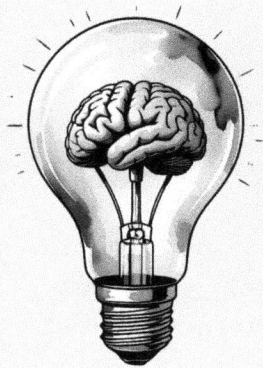

Making Sense Of It
The Nature of Shock After Miscarriage

Shock is one of the body's oldest survival strategies. When a devastating loss hits — like a miscarriage — your nervous system doesn't always rush straight into grief. Instead, it often puts up a kind of shield. You may feel detached, stunned, or like you're walking through your life from outside your own body. Some people describe it as being underwater. Others say it's as though the world kept spinning while they were frozen in place. None of these reactions mean you don't care or aren't grieving "the right way." They mean your body is giving you temporary scaffolding to survive the collapse of what you expected.

Psychologists explain that shock is your system's way of slowing down what would otherwise be an unbearable flood of emotion. The numbness you may feel is not failure — it's protection. And yet, this protection can come with confusion. You might wonder, Why am I not crying more? Why can I still go to work? Why do I feel so hollow instead of falling apart? These are not signs that you are broken — they are signs that you are human.

What makes miscarriage grief uniquely disorienting is how invisible it often is. In most cultures, miscarriage rarely comes with the rituals or collective acknowledgement that follow other losses. There is no funeral program, no gathering where people hold your hand and say, I'm so sorry for your loss. Instead, silence surrounds you. Sociologists note that this silence deepens the shock, because loss without recognition leaves the griever stranded in what feels like an alternate reality — something life-changing has happened, yet the world refuses to reflect it back to you.

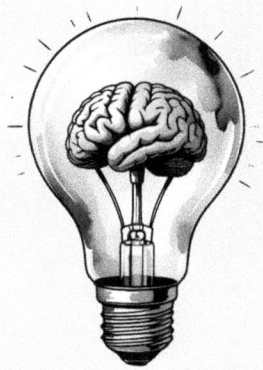

Making Sense Of It
The Nature of Shock After Miscarriage

Anthropologists who study grief across cultures find that in communities where miscarriage is honored through shared ritual — whether through naming ceremonies, candles, or gatherings — women report lower feelings of shame and alienation. What this tells us is profound: shock is not only biological, it's relational. Humans are wired to metabolize loss together, but miscarriage often forces people into solitude. You may be carrying both the private ache of what your body has gone through and the public ache of being unseen.

And then there is the matter of identity. Even in early pregnancy, many people begin weaving a story — imagining names, futures, family roles. When miscarriage interrupts that story, the shock isn't just about physical loss; it's about the collapse of a narrative you had already begun to live inside. That collapse can feel like falling through a trapdoor with nothing to hold onto.

So if you find yourself stunned, numb, or floating through your days as though the ground is unstable, know this: you are not failing at grief. You are living through its first stage — the mind and body's attempt to keep you intact long enough to eventually face what has happened. The numbness, the disbelief, the hollow space inside you — these are the marks of shock, not the measure of your love. Naming this is the beginning of making space for your healing.

What did your body feel like when you first learned of the miscarriage?

Take a moment to close your eyes and reflect on that moment. How did your body respond — tension, numbness, or a sense of emptiness? What emotions did you notice in your body but couldn't put into words? Write whatever comes to mind, even if it doesn't make sense yet.

What did your body feel like when you first learned of the miscarriage?

What did you believe or hope for before this loss?

Before the miscarriage, what were your hopes for the pregnancy or your future as a parent? What dreams and expectations did you have that now feel like they've been taken from you? Write down the thoughts that surface, and be gentle with yourself as you acknowledge what was lost.

What did you believe or hope for before this loss?

How do you feel about your grief right now?

Often, grief doesn't show up in clear, understandable ways. How are you feeling right now? Confused? Disconnected? Maybe you feel numb or detached. Reflect on the emotions you're feeling and give yourself permission to not have to make sense of everything just yet.

How do you feel about your grief right now?

What is one word that describes your current emotional state?

Sometimes we can't articulate the full depth of our grief, but there may be a word that feels closest to what you're experiencing. It could be something like "empty," "heavy," "numb," or "lost." Whatever it is, write about why that word feels fitting, and let yourself sit with it.

What is one word that describes your current emotional state?

How can you offer yourself compassion during this time of shock?

When we're in shock, we often forget to care for ourselves in the way we need. What is one small act of kindness you can offer yourself today? Perhaps it's resting, allowing yourself to cry, or simply acknowledging that it's okay not to be okay. Write about what self-compassion looks like for you right now.

How can you offer yourself compassion during this time of shock?

TRACING THE TRUTH

THE RIPPLE MAP

When something as sudden as miscarriage happens, the shock doesn't stay in one place — it ripples through your body, your relationships, even the way you see yourself. This exercise gives you a way to gently map out those ripples so you can see them more clearly, instead of carrying them as a blur inside you.

Why it helps:
Shock scatters experiences, making it hard to see the whole picture. Mapping the ripples brings order to chaos. It lets you step back and see your grief not as "all of me" but as waves touching different parts of life — waves that can eventually settle.

Label each circle with a part of life touched by this loss: My body, My emotions, My relationships, My sense of self, My future plans.
In each ripple, write short words or phrases about what feels altered. For example:
My body: "empty, disconnected, confused"
My relationships: "don't know how to talk about it"
My future plans: "suddenly unclear"

TRACING THE TRUTH

THE RIPPLE MAP

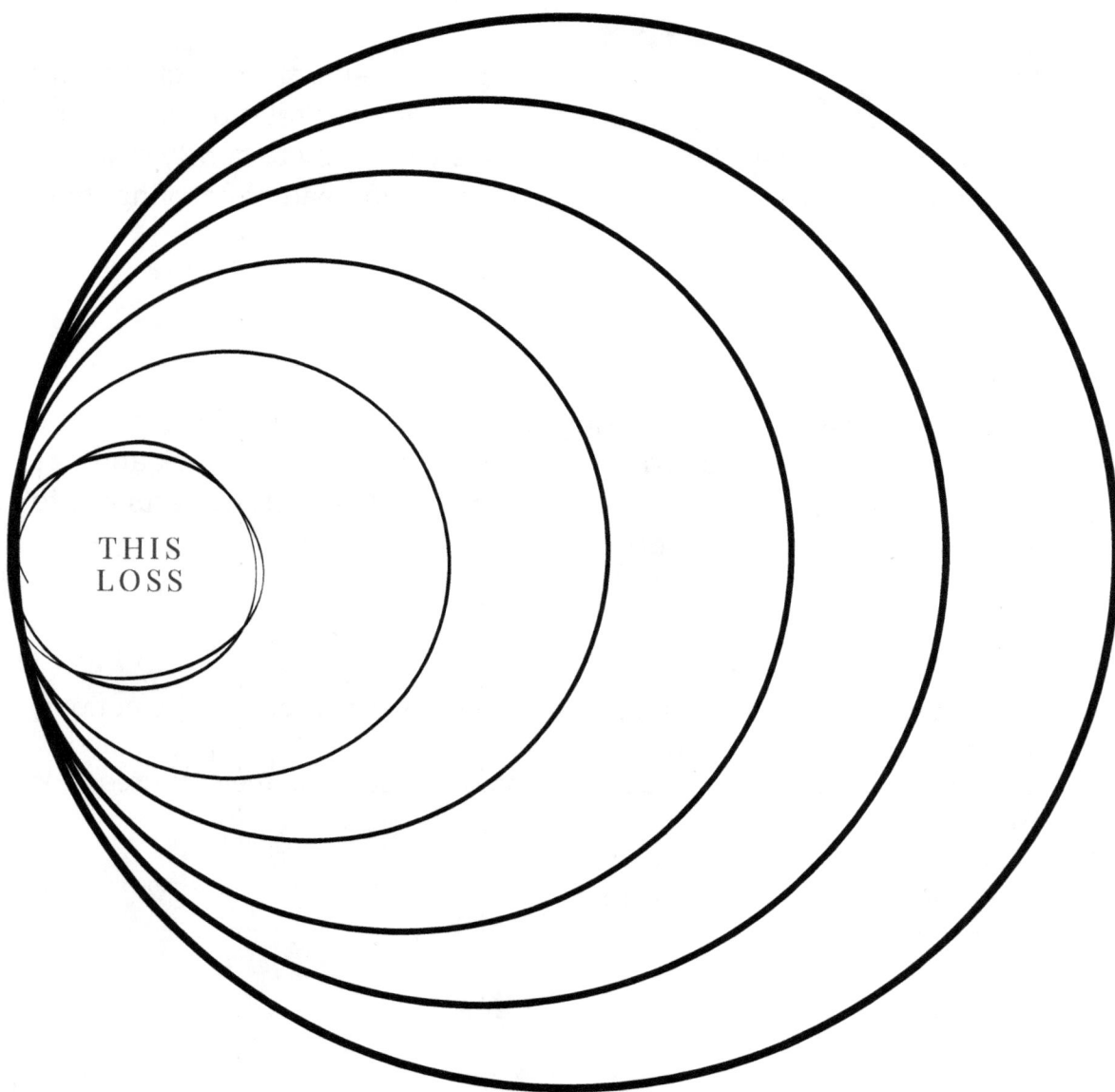

THIS
LOSS

TRACING THE TRUTH

THE INTERRUPTED STORY

Every pregnancy begins to write a story — sometimes quietly, sometimes with vivid detail. Miscarriage interrupts that story mid-sentence, leaving you holding fragments that feel impossible to piece together. This exercise invites you to lay those fragments down with honesty and care, creating space for what was imagined and for what was lost.

Why it helps:
Shock often comes from an unfinished story — your mind was already weaving meaning, and then the narrative cut off mid-sentence. Putting those pieces on paper acknowledges the rupture while also creating space for a future chapter, whenever you're ready.

Write two paragraphs:
- **Paragraph One: The Story I Was Beginning to Tell.** Describe what you were picturing — even if it was just starting. Hopes, names, small details, or the feeling of expectation.
- **Paragraph Two: The Story That Stopped Suddenly.** Write about the moment it changed — how it ended, what disappeared, and what silence followed.

- **Leave space for a third paragraph** you'll return to later in the workbook: The Story I Am Still Living. You don't need to write it now. Just mark the space.

TRACING THE TRUTH

THE INTERRUPTED STORY

TRACING THE TRUTH

THE INTERRUPTED STORY

MAPPING YOUR RESILIENCE

When life is painful, the spotlight lands on what's broken or lost. But every hard season you've lived through also carries evidence of your resilience. Mapping your past with a "strength lens" helps you reclaim those forgotten skills — endurance, creativity, boundary-setting, persistence, humor, or compassion. Trauma research shows that naming and revisiting these strengths rebuilds self-trust. Instead of seeing your past only as a string of wounds, you begin to recognize the ways you showed up for yourself. Circling three core strengths creates a personal toolkit you can consciously bring forward into your next chapter.

1 **Draw Your Timeline** —Mark a few "hard seasons" you've lived through on the timeline.

2 **Name Strengths** — Under each event, write one or two strengths you used to get through (e.g., courage, asking for help, persistence).

3 **Circle Three** — Look at the whole map. Circle three strengths that feel most alive, relevant, or needed for where you're headed now.

4 **Carry Them Forward** — Write them on a sticky note or card where you'll see them often — reminders that you've done hard things before, and you will again.

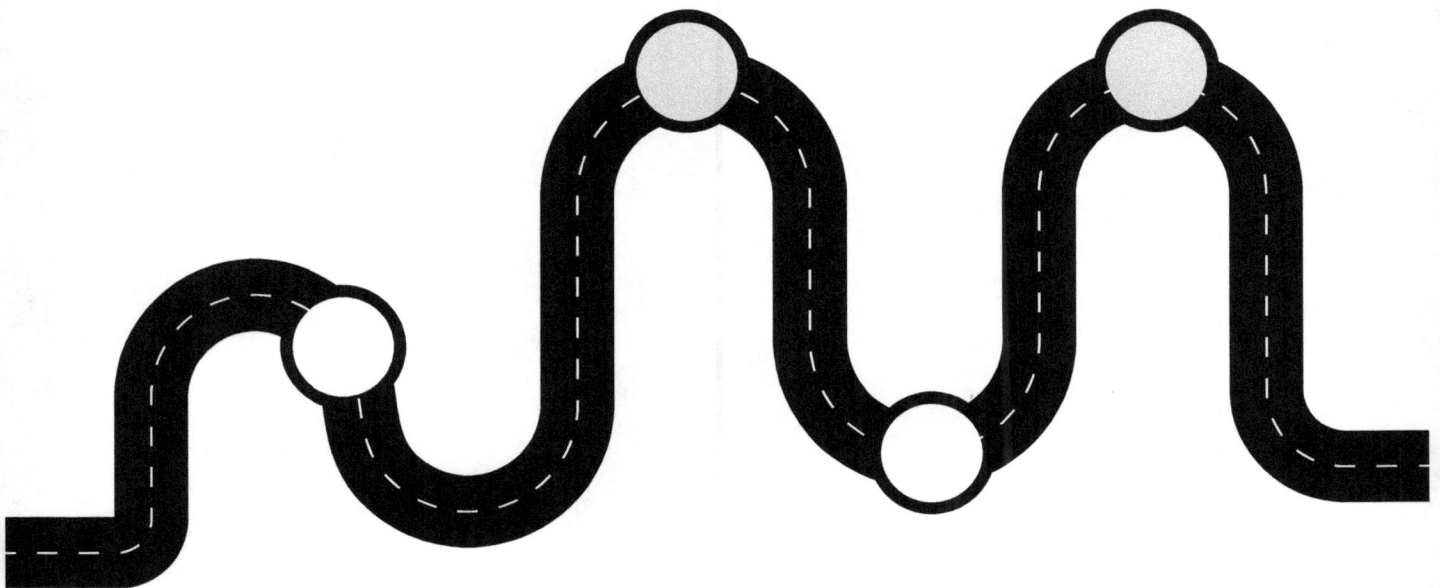

SAFE/BRAVE COLLAGE

Healing doesn't mean throwing yourself into the deep end. It means finding the edges of your current safety and gently stretching them. This exercise blends comfort and courage, showing your nervous system that bravery doesn't have to mean danger. Visual imagery (like collage) activates deeper parts of the brain than words alone, helping you bypass self-criticism and connect with possibility. Placing one "brave" image inside your "safe" space signals: I can grow without abandoning myself. This balance between grounding and stretching is key for trauma recovery, resilience, and lasting change.

Collect Images — Use magazines, printouts, or sketches. On the Safe side, paste images that represent rest, comfort, and security. On the Brave side, add images that symbolize courage, growth, or edges you dream of touching.

The Bridge Step — Choose one tiny image of bravery and place it into the Safe half. This represents your next gentle edge — a stretch that doesn't abandon your grounding.

Reflect — Ask yourself: What's one small way I can practice this edge this wee

SAFE   BRAVE

EMOTIONS IN COLOR

Emotions can feel abstract or overwhelming when we only experience them as "stress" or "sadness." Adding color and body mapping turns them into something tangible, something you can see, name, and notice. This makes emotional awareness less scary and more approachable. By shading intensity and locating the sensations in your body, you start to recognize patterns, triggers, and areas that need extra care. This is not about judging the feeling — it's about mapping your internal landscape so you can respond with awareness rather than autopilot. Over time, it builds clarity, emotional literacy, and the ability to intervene with skillful action before overwhelm takes over.

Pick Colors — Assign a color to each emotion that feels right for you.
Shade Intensity — Color each wedge to reflect how strongly you feel that emotion today.
Body Mapping — Next to the wheel, jot where in your body each emotion lives (chest tightness, stomach flutter, jaw tension).
Reflect — Notice patterns, imbalances, or surprises. Consider one small action to soothe or honor a strong area.

SECTION TWO

Grieving the Unseen – Acknowledging the Loss That Can't Be Held

Miscarriage is a grief that's hard to articulate, especially when the life you lost is still so small, so unseen. There's no baby to mourn in your arms, no memorial or funeral to mark the end. It can feel like the grief is invisible — something you feel deeply but can't always show the world. This type of grief is profoundly lonely at times, as the loss might not feel "real" to others because they can't see it. But it is real, and it is yours. The loss of what could have been, of what was starting to take shape in your heart and mind, is deeply valid and deserving of your grief. In this section, we will explore the concept of grieving something unseen, something intangible. It's a process that often brings up conflicting emotions, from guilt or shame to anger and despair.

You might feel like your grief is minimized because others don't understand, or because society places so little value on the loss of a pregnancy. But this is a profound loss, and your emotions, however they appear, are important. We'll also talk about how to embrace this invisible grief, find its language, and begin to honor it.

38

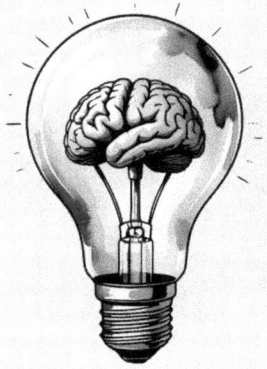

Making Sense Of It
The Weight of Invisible Grief

One of the most painful truths about miscarriage is that the grief often has no outward marker. In other losses, there are rituals that make pain visible — funerals, memorials, sympathy cards, casseroles brought by neighbors. These rituals act as both mirrors and containers, reflecting grief back to the mourner and holding some of its weight. But with miscarriage, those rituals rarely exist. There is no baby blanket to fold away, no eulogy spoken aloud, no official moment when the world pauses to say, Something precious was lost here. The silence around it can leave you feeling suspended, carrying a sorrow that has nowhere to land.

Psychologists describe this as disenfranchised grief — grief that society does not fully recognize. When your grief is invisible to others, you may start to question its legitimacy yourself. You may hear a voice inside whispering, It was early. Maybe it doesn't count. Maybe I'm making too much of this. But grief does not measure itself by gestational weeks or by whether others acknowledge your loss. Grief measures itself by attachment — the bond you were already forming, the identity you were beginning to inhabit, the visions of a future you had already started to imagine. That bond was real. That future mattered. And so does your grief.

Sociologists note that invisible grief carries a double burden: not only the ache of the loss itself, but also the loneliness of not being seen in it. This can make you feel split in two — holding a storm inside while outwardly functioning as though life is unchanged. It is profoundly human to long for someone to bear witness, to say, I see what you lost, even if I can't touch it.

40

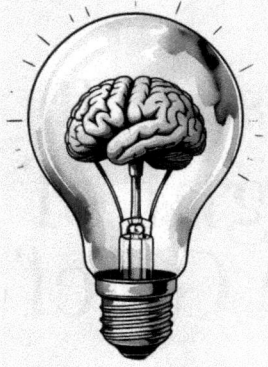

Making Sense Of It
The Weight of Invisible Grief

Anthropologists who study mourning across cultures have found that when communities create rituals for pregnancy loss — whether through naming ceremonies, planting trees, or shared storytelling — those who grieve report less shame, less isolation, and a stronger sense of continuity. This shows us something vital: loss does not need to be tangible to be worthy of ritual. Humans have always needed ways to anchor sorrow in the physical world, to take what feels invisible and make it known.

Without those anchors, grief can float untethered, leaving you unsure how to process it.

This unseen grief also collides with your identity. Many people begin to step into the role of parent long before birth. They may talk to their baby, picture their face, or imagine holding them. When miscarriage ends that story, you may feel stripped of an identity you had already started to wear. You might find yourself asking, Was I ever really a parent? Do I still count? These questions live at the intersection of love and erasure, and they can be some of the most painful to carry alone.

And yet, here is the truth: your grief is real, even if others cannot see it. The absence of a body to hold does not erase the presence of love. The lack of ceremony does not mean your loss deserves silence. This grief may be invisible to the outside world, but within you, it is valid, sacred, and deserving of space. The act of naming what is unseen — of giving words, rituals, or meaning to what was lost — is not only healing, it is a quiet act of reclamation. It is a way of saying this mattered.

What is the thing you are grieving, even though no one else can see it?

Take a moment to reflect on what feels lost to you. What are you mourning that can't be physically held? It might be the dreams, the hopes, or the future you imagined with this pregnancy. Write about the unseen loss that is uniquely yours, without concern for how others might view it.

What is the thing you are grieving, even though no one else can see it?

How has your grief been invisible to others, and how does that make you feel?

Many who experience miscarriage feel a sense of invisibility or invalidation. Reflect on how your grief has been overlooked or misunderstood by those around you. What does that bring up for you emotionally? Is there anger, sadness, or a feeling of isolation? Allow yourself to explore these feelings.

How has your grief been invisible to others, and how does that make you feel?

What would you say to others if you could help them understand your loss?

Sometimes, it's hard to put into words the depth of a loss that others cannot see. Imagine explaining your grief to someone who has not experienced miscarriage. What would you want them to understand? Write down everything you would say, even if it feels hard to express.

What would you say to others if you could help them understand your loss?

What do you wish you could have done to "hold" this loss?

Grieving the unseen often leaves us feeling powerless. Reflect on what you feel you missed out on — a ritual, a moment, an action — that could have symbolized your grief. Write about what you wish you could have done to acknowledge or "hold" this loss in a tangible way.

What do you wish you could have done to "hold" this loss?

What would it mean to acknowledge your grief as just as real as any other loss?

So often, we downplay grief when there is no physical object to mourn. Write about what it would feel like to give yourself permission to fully acknowledge this loss as real and significant, without minimizing or dismissing it. How does that change how you see yourself and your grief?

What would it mean to acknowledge your grief as just as real as any other loss?

TRACING THE TRUTH

THE EMPTY SPACE LETTER

Even though there's no one to hold, your grief still exists, and it deserves recognition. This exercise gives you a safe space to speak to the life you lost — to name your love, your sorrow, and the dreams that never had a chance to bloom.

Why it helps:
Writing a letter makes the unseen visible. It anchors grief in language, giving you a container for feelings that otherwise float unspoken. It creates a witness — even if the only witness is the page.

On a blank page, write a short letter addressed to the one you lost.
Begin with something like: "Even though I cannot hold you, I want you to know..." and allow your words to flow.
You might write about the dreams you had, the love you felt, the ache of not getting to meet them. Keep it raw, imperfect, and honest.

TRACING THE TRUTH

THE EMPTY SPACE LETTER

---.

---.

---.

---.

---.

---.

---.

---.

---.

---.

---.

---.

---.

---53

TRACING THE TRUTH

THE EMPTY SPACE LETTER

TRACING THE TRUTH

THE EMPTY SPACE LETTER

TRACING THE TRUTH

CREATING A RITUAL OF REMEMBRANCE

Sometimes grief needs a quiet, tangible space to live in — a moment that belongs entirely to your loss. This simple ritual gives form to what is unseen, honoring the life you imagined and the love you already carried, even if only in your heart.

Why it helps:
Creating a ritual helps give structure and meaning to your grief. It allows you to symbolize the loss in a tangible way, even though there is no physical baby to hold. This can help you feel that your grief is seen and acknowledged, even if it's invisible to others.

Choose a meaningful object or symbol that you can use in your ritual. It could be a candle, a stone, a flower, or anything that feels symbolic to you. The goal is to find something that can represent the pregnancy or what it might have become.

Find a quiet space where you can sit alone. This could be in nature, your home, or a place that feels peaceful.

Light the candle or place the object on a flat surface in front of you. As you do so, say aloud (or in your mind), "This is to honor what was lost — the dreams, the future, the baby I never got to hold."

Spend a few minutes in silence, allowing any feelings to arise. There is no rush here; let your emotions come without trying to control them. If tears come, let them flow. If you feel numb, sit with that too.

THREE PILLARS BEFORE NOON

When you're caught in anxiety, depression, or burnout, your nervous system can swing between shutdown and overdrive. The quickest way to steady yourself is to touch three key areas: body, mind, and pleasure. Moving your body brings energy online; completing a mastery task (even something small like an email) restores a sense of competence; and engaging in pleasure reminds you that joy and safety are still accessible. This "trio" isn't about being productive — it's about balance. Think of it as a daily reset button. By noon, if you've already touched your body, completed one mastery task, and tasted one moment of pleasure, you've laid down anchors for resilience. Instead of asking your day to be perfect, you give yourself three touchpoints that prove: I can show up, I can accomplish, and I can enjoy.

Body: Pick one simple movement (walk, stretch, yoga, dancing in your kitchen).

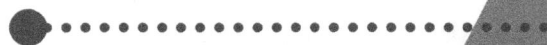

Mastery: Choose one achievable task that gives a sense of completion (send an email, pay a bill, tidy a corner).

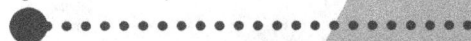

Pleasure: Select one thing that nourishes (listen to music, sip tea, step into sunlight).

Stack them early: Aim to complete all three before noon to set your rhythm.

Reflect briefly: Notice how touching all three domains shifts your mood and energy.

MOOD MAPPING BY THE HOUR

Our mood is never random — it's deeply influenced by what we do, when we do it, and how our nervous system responds. When depression or anxiety is heavy, it can feel like nothing makes a difference. This log helps you prove to yourself that even small activities shift your emotional state, sometimes by just one point. And that one-point lift matters — it's momentum, a reminder that you aren't stuck forever. By tracking your mood alongside your activities, you build a personalized map of what nourishes you. Instead of relying on guesswork, you'll have hard evidence of your own resilience patterns. Over time, this practice shows you that certain choices (a call with a safe friend, a walk outside, finishing a task) consistently bring relief. This isn't about forcing happiness — it's about noticing what gently nudges you toward better.

For one day, each hour, write down what you're doing and your mood (0–10).

Repeat for a few days — notice patterns.

Circle activities that reliably lift you by at least one point.

Intentionally schedule more of those "one-point lifts" into your week.

Revisit the log whenever you feel stuck, to remind yourself you have options.

Day	Activity	Mood Before	Mood After

MOOD MAPPING BY THE HOUR

Day	Activity	Mood Before	Mood After

SECTION THREE

The Weight of Silence – Navigating Expectations and Conversations After Loss

When you first experience a miscarriage, the grief can feel like an overwhelming wave — a deep, hollow sensation that strikes unexpectedly. You might have been planning, dreaming, or even just beginning to get excited, and in an instant, everything changes. The shock can be paralyzing. It might feel like you're suspended in time, unable to fully grasp the magnitude of what's happening, yet deeply aware of the loss.

This section is here to sit with you in that moment of confusion and disorientation. Grief is often not a linear path, and the shock of miscarriage can leave you feeling numb, disbelieving, or even distant from your own emotions. It's okay to feel like your world has suddenly tilted, as though you're struggling to find your footing. The purpose here is not to rush through the pain but to give yourself permission to feel what you need to feel, without judgment. It's natural to wonder if you'll ever feel "normal" again, or if the weight of this loss will always haunt you. What's important is to recognize that your body, mind, and heart are beginning a process of deep healing — even if it doesn't feel like it right now. In this section, we'll explore how shock can manifest in both your body and mind, and begin to create a space where healing can slowly take root.

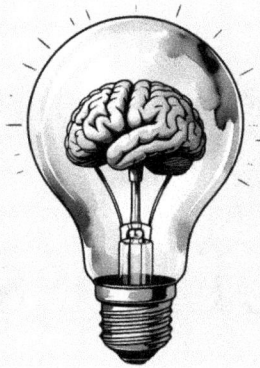

Making Sense Of It
The Ripple Effect of Loss

Miscarriage doesn't exist in a vacuum. While the loss is deeply personal, it radiates outward, touching every connection in your life. Friends, family, and partners can feel the tremor of grief too — but often in ways that leave you feeling alone. Their discomfort, their silence, or even their attempts to "fix" things can make you feel unseen, misunderstood, or emotionally stranded. Sometimes silence can sting like a betrayal, not because your loved ones are uncaring, but because grief is uncomfortable and most people simply don't know how to bear witness to it.

Partners often grieve differently. One might retreat into quiet reflection or focus on practicalities, while the other feels raw, urgent, and uncontainable emotion. These differences can feel like distance, creating a painful gap at a time when connection is desperately needed. Friends may offer clichés, reassurances, or "solutions" that inadvertently minimize your experience. Family members may expect you to "move on" or to return to normalcy on their timeline. Sociologically, miscarriage grief is layered with cultural scripts that define what is appropriate to feel, how long to grieve, and which losses count. All of this can compound isolation, leaving you to navigate an invisible, unacknowledged weight almost entirely on your own.

Within this relational landscape, boundaries are not just helpful — they are essential. They are a declaration that your grief matters, that your emotional wellbeing deserves protection, and that you are allowed to control the terms of engagement with others.

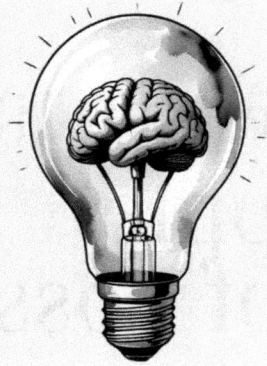

Making Sense Of It
The Ripple Effect of Loss

Boundaries might mean saying, I need space right now, or, Please don't offer advice unless I ask for it. They might look like choosing carefully whom you speak to about the loss, or deciding when and how to participate in family gatherings, social events, or conversations about pregnancy. Boundaries are not walls of isolation; they are scaffolding, giving your heart and nervous system a safe container to process grief.

From a psychological perspective, this process also restores agency in a time when power often feels stolen. Miscarriage can leave you feeling powerless — over your body, your plans, and even your narrative. Establishing boundaries is one of the few ways to reclaim control. It signals to yourself and the world that your grief is valid, that your body and mind require respect, and that healing cannot be rushed or forced to fit someone else's expectations.

Grief, especially when compounded by relational misunderstanding, is messy. You may feel anger, sadness, resentment, and confusion all at once — sometimes toward yourself, sometimes toward others. These feelings are not wrong. They are part of the human response to a loss that is invisible, yet profound. Recognizing the social and relational dimensions of your grief allows you to name not only what you lost, but also the ways the loss has reverberated through your connections.

This awareness is transformative. By observing how grief moves through relationships, identifying patterns of misunderstanding, and setting protective boundaries, you create a space where mourning can exist fully. You teach your nervous system that it is safe to feel, and you communicate to the people around you — consciously or unconsciously — that your emotions are valid.

How have others responded to your loss?

Reflect on how the people in your life have reacted to your miscarriage. Have they acknowledged your grief, avoided it, or tried to minimize it? Write about the ways people have communicated (or failed to communicate) with you, and how that made you feel.

How have others responded to your loss?

What expectations from others feel most difficult to carry?

Sometimes people have unspoken expectations — that you should be "okay" after a certain amount of time, or that you should be "strong" for others. Think about any unspoken or explicit expectations you've felt after your miscarriage. How have they impacted your healing?

What expectations from others feel most difficult to carry?

What is your biggest need right now in terms of emotional support?

Take some time to reflect on what would feel most helpful to you in terms of support. What do you wish people would understand about what you need — whether it's silence, a shoulder to cry on, or simply someone to listen without offering solutions? Write about the kind of support you crave and why it's important for your healing.

What is your biggest need right now in terms of emotional support?

How do you want to navigate conversations about your miscarriage with others?

Talking about your loss can be difficult, especially when you're uncertain of how others will react. Write about how you would like these conversations to unfold. What do you need to say, and how can you communicate your grief to others in a way that feels safe for you?

How do you want to navigate conversations about your miscarriage with others?

What is your experience with avoiding or silencing your own grief?

Sometimes, we can become complicit in silencing our grief to avoid discomfort or judgment from others. Reflect on how you've responded to your own grief in social settings. Have you minimized it or avoided talking about it? Explore why this happens and what would be required for you to stop silencing your grief.

What is your experience with avoiding or silencing your own grief?

TRACING THE TRUTH

MAPPING YOUR
EMOTIONAL LANDSCAPE

Your inner clarity is the best guide for what you can tolerate and what you cannot. This exercise links reflection with somatic awareness.

Why it helps:
Seeing your relational map allows you to step back from the emotional fog. It helps identify which connections amplify your grief and which offer support, giving clarity to how to navigate them.

Around the circle, draw smaller circles for key relationships (partner, friends, family, coworkers).

Draw lines connecting your grief circle to each relationship circle. On each line, write a few words describing how your grief interacts with that person — for example: "feels unseen," "they try to fix me," "creates tension," or "I feel comforted."

Notice patterns. Are there relationships that feel supportive? Ones that feel draining? Ones that are both?

TRACING THE TRUTH

MAPPING YOUR EMOTIONAL LANDSCAPE

ME & MY
GRIEF

TRACING THE TRUTH

BOUNDARY BLUEPRINT

Protecting your emotional space is an essential part of healing. This exercise gives you a clear, simple way to identify and communicate the boundaries you need with the people around you.

Why it helps:
This exercise makes boundaries concrete. Writing them down transforms vague feelings of overwhelm into actionable steps, helping you protect your nervous system and grief process.

Fill in each row with a person or group you interact with.
For Boundary Needed, write what you need to protect your emotional space (e.g., "I need them to avoid giving advice" or "I need to leave the room if pregnancy is discussed").
In the last column, write down how you will communicate it in a calm, clear way. It can be as simple as: "I appreciate your care, but I need to process this in my own time."

TRACING THE TRUTH

BOUNDARY BLUEPRINT

Relationship	Boundary Needed	How I Will Communicate It

SELF-COMPASSION BREAK

When stress, shame, or pain flare up, most of us go straight into self-criticism: Why can't I handle this better? What's wrong with me? That inner attack only tightens the spiral. Kristin Neff's Self-Compassion Break interrupts that cycle. It gives you three small handholds: recognition of your pain, the reminder you're not alone in it, and an active choice to soften instead of harden against yourself. With repetition, your nervous system learns that you don't have to white-knuckle through suffering or numb out — you can meet yourself with the same tenderness you'd extend to a friend. That shift doesn't erase the pain, but it changes the way it lands in your body. Over time, it builds resilience, because you're no longer abandoned in hard moments; you become your own safe ally.

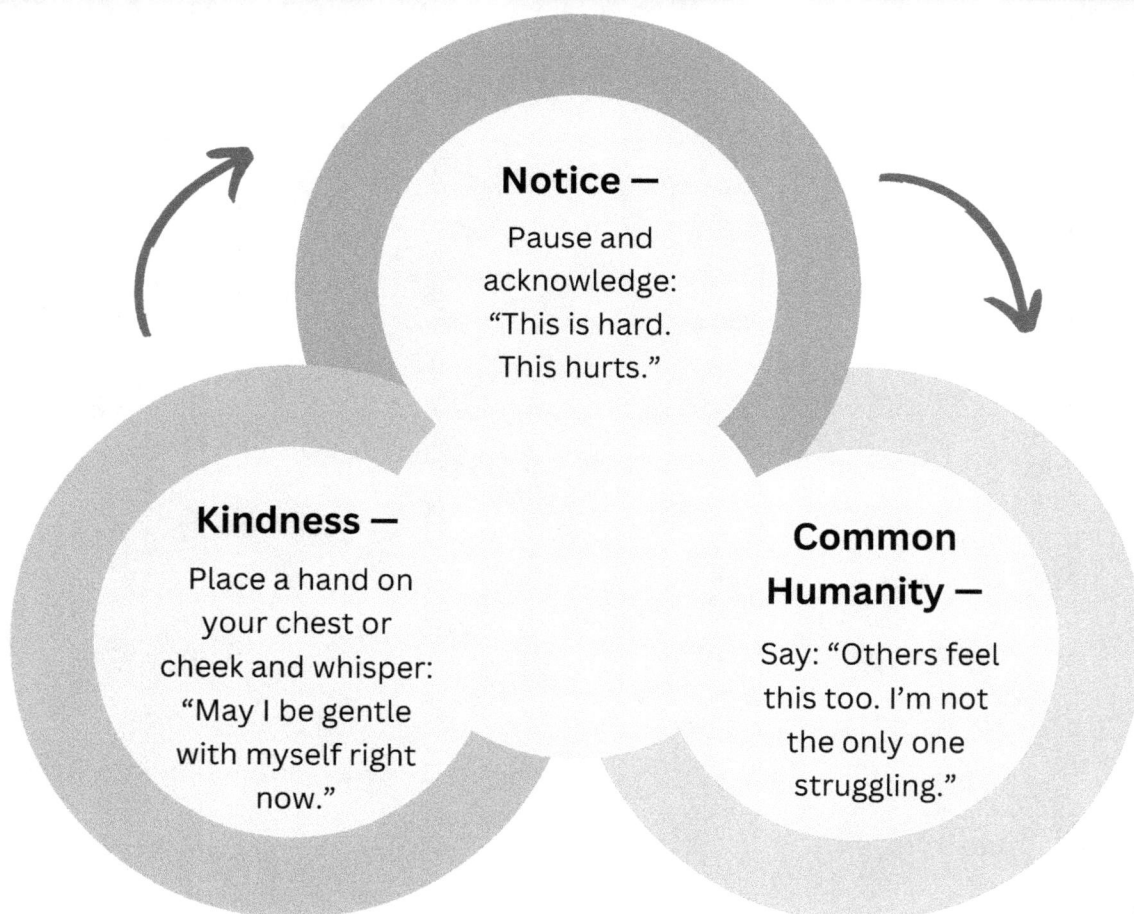

Notice —
Pause and acknowledge: "This is hard. This hurts."

Kindness —
Place a hand on your chest or cheek and whisper: "May I be gentle with myself right now."

Common Humanity —
Say: "Others feel this too. I'm not the only one struggling."

POCKET MOOD LIFTERS

When life feels heavy, it's easy to forget what actually helps. In hard moments, the brain tends to focus on what's wrong, not what's available. An Antidote List is your preloaded reminder: ten small, proven things that shift your state even a little. These aren't grand fixes or instant cures — they're micro-adjustments that keep you from sliding deeper into the stuckness. Pairing an antidote before a hard task helps you face it with steadier energy; using one after provides recovery and closure so you don't carry the weight forward. Over time, this list becomes muscle memory — your nervous system learns, When I struggle, I have options. That's the opposite of hopelessness.

1 **List Ten** — Write down 10 things that reliably lift your mood (a song, a walk, fresh air, texting a safe friend, lighting a candle). Keep them small and doable.

....

....

....

....

....

....

....

....

2 **Use Before** — Pick one before facing a task you tend to dread. Let it soften resistance.

3 **Use After** — Choose another as a closing ritual. Let it tell your body, That part is done. I'm safe again.

SECTION FOUR

Blaming My Body – Shame, Guilt, and the Physicality of Loss

After a miscarriage, many people find themselves caught in a quiet war with their own bodies. You might wonder: What went wrong? What did I do? Why couldn't my body hold on? These thoughts aren't just passing fears — they become shame-laced echoes that can live in your muscles, breath, and bones. Even when doctors offer rational explanations, your emotional brain might whisper, I failed. It can feel like your body betrayed you, and for some, like you betrayed the baby.

This section is about making space for the painful intersection between grief and embodiment — where loss is felt not only emotionally but physically. We'll explore the somatic experience of miscarriage grief, the internalized shame it often brings, and how to gently begin the process of repairing your relationship with your body. You are not broken. Your body is not your enemy. Let's begin to soften the blame and offer your body the compassion it deserves.

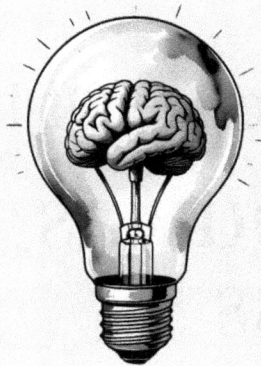

Making Sense Of It
The Body as Witness

Miscarriage can leave you feeling like your body has turned against you. That sensation — of betrayal, failure, or inadequacy — is not uncommon, and it is deeply human. Psychologically, this response is tied to the way our brains process loss and self-perception. When something as profound as pregnancy ends prematurely, the mind often searches for a cause, a point of control. In the absence of answers, many people turn inward, asking, Was it something I did? Could I have prevented this? This internalized questioning can quickly spiral into shame, guilt, and self-blame.

Neuroscience tells us that the brain does not distinguish sharply between emotional and physical pain. The grief you feel emotionally manifests in your body — tight shoulders, constricted chest, shallow breath, or an ache in your stomach. Shame and guilt, in particular, are embodied experiences. They lodge in muscle tension, posture, and even movement patterns, silently reminding you of the perceived "failure" each day. This is why miscarriage grief can feel heavy, relentless, and physical — your body is literally carrying the loss with you.

Sociologically, our culture amplifies these pressures. Society often treats miscarriage as an invisible or "lesser" loss, subtly suggesting that it shouldn't leave a mark or that you shouldn't grieve too loudly. Those cultural messages reinforce the idea that the body should be "efficient," that it failed, or that your worth is tied to reproductive outcomes. This messaging can worsen the internalized shame, making you question your body's reliability and your own value.

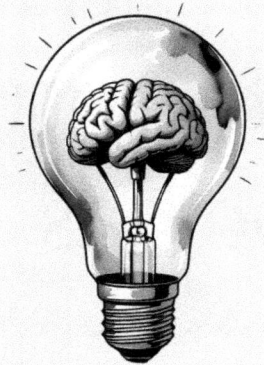

Making Sense Of It
The Body as Witness

Anthropologically, cultures that ritualize pregnancy loss — through ceremonies, memorials, or somatic practices — show the opposite effect. Acknowledging the body's role, honoring its efforts, and giving grief a physical and communal container allows people to release both emotional and embodied tension. In contrast, when loss is silenced, the body often becomes the silent repository of guilt, shame, and sorrow.

The path to healing begins with reclaiming your body as an ally, not an enemy. This means noticing the tension in your muscles without judgment, breathing into spaces where shame lingers, and offering conscious compassion to your physical self. Your body carried life, however briefly, and endured a profound loss. It is not a traitor — it is a witness, a vessel of experience, and a partner in your healing. By listening to your body, naming the guilt and shame it has absorbed, and responding with gentleness, you begin to repair the relationship that miscarriage may have fractured.

You are not broken. The physical ache and emotional weight you carry are natural responses to an unnatural event. With patience and care, your body can become a source of grounding, solace, and resilience — reminding you that grief is real, embodied, and worthy of acknowledgment, but that it does not define your worth or your future.

What have you believed about your body since your miscarriage?

Reflect on the inner dialogue you've had with or about your body. Has it been kind, cruel, confused, or disconnected? Bring awareness to the tone and content of how you relate to your physical self in this season of grief.

What have you believed about your body since your miscarriage?

Do you feel a sense of betrayal, guilt, or blame toward your body?

If so, allow yourself to write freely and honestly. What are the accusations you haven't said out loud? Putting them on the page doesn't mean they're true — it just gives them space to breathe so they don't fester in silence.

Do you feel a sense of betrayal, guilt, or blame toward your body?

In what ways has your body tried to protect or support you during this time?

Think about how your body has carried your grief, your endurance, and your attempts at healing. What sensations, instincts, or somatic memories rise as you reflect on your body not as a betrayer, but as a witness?

In what ways has your body tried to protect or support you during this time?

What have you lost in your relationship with your body — and what would you like to reclaim?

Has your sense of embodiment, femininity, fertility, or safety shifted? This is a tender space — reflect on what feels lost and what kind of relationship you long to rebuild with your body.

What have you lost in your relationship with your body — and what would you like to reclaim?

What would compassion toward your body look like today?

Not forever — just today. Would it look like rest? A warm bath? Touching your belly with kindness instead of blame? Allow yourself to imagine one small act of softness you could offer yourself.

What would compassion toward your body look like today?

If your body could speak to you, what might it say?

Imagine that your body has its own voice — one that is wise, patient, and burdened in its own way. What would it say about what it's been through, and what it needs from you now?

If your body could speak to you, what might it say?

MY SAFETY NET

In moments of overwhelm, your nervous system isn't wired to pause and think through options — it leaps into fight, flight, or freeze. A written safety plan is like a ready-made anchor: instead of spiraling or going blank, you have a clear map back to calm. By identifying your unique triggers, early warning signs, and support network ahead of time, you create a sense of control and reassurance. This is less about predicting every crisis and more about telling your body and mind: I have a way back.

Identify triggers: Write down situations, phrases, or tones of voice that tend to spark distress.

Notice early warning signs: List how your body tells you stress is rising (racing heart, clenched jaw, shallow breath).

Choose three rapid-calm skills: Breathing, grounding, or movement tools you can use quickly.

Name two safe people: Write their contact info. Keep the plan somewhere visible or carry a copy with you.

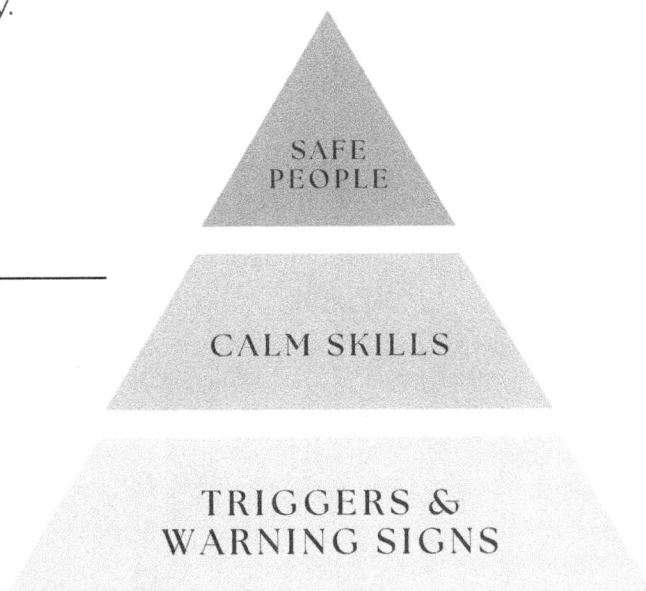

SAFE PEOPLE

CALM SKILLS

TRIGGERS & WARNING SIGNS

WINDOW OF TOLERANCE MAP

When you're dysregulated — whether spun up with racing thoughts or shut down and numb — it's almost impossible to think clearly. Mapping your "window of tolerance" gives you a visual reminder of what your nervous system looks and feels like when it's balanced, overstimulated, or under-engaged. Instead of feeling hijacked, you can recognize: "Ah, I'm outside my window right now." That awareness alone widens your choices. It also keeps you from turning regulation into a guessing game; you'll have a personal roadmap of cues and tools that work for you.

Fill in personal cues. For each state, jot what you notice in your body, thoughts, and emotions. (Example: Hyper = clenched jaw, racing mind. Hypo = heavy limbs, flat affect.)

Add regulation tools. Next to Hyper, write 2–3 down-regulating skills (ex: slow breathing, grounding). Next to Hypo, add up-regulating ones (ex: movement, music).

Calm/Present (your window)	Hyper (revved-up)	Hypo (shut-down)

Regulation Tools

POCKET OF SAFETY

When stress hits, your nervous system automatically searches for threat. Resource installation interrupts that loop by giving your body a felt reminder of safety, strength, or care. Instead of only rehearsing pain, you practice anchoring to something nurturing and stabilizing. This isn't about pretending the hard stuff doesn't exist — it's about teaching your brain and body that safety and support also exist. By pairing the memory with a body cue (like placing your hand on your heart), you create a portable anchor you can return to whenever you feel unsteady. Over time, this strengthens your capacity to self-soothe and widen your window of tolerance.

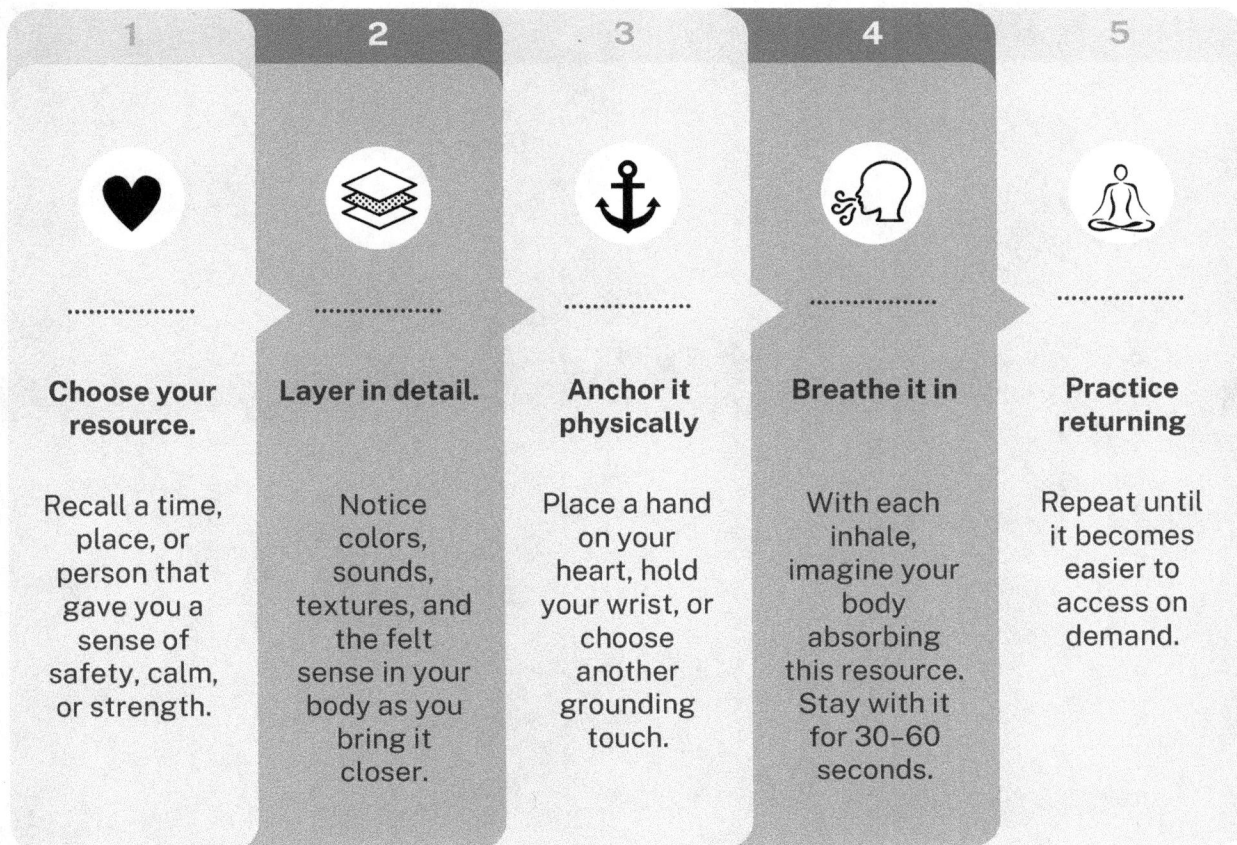

1	2	3	4	5
Choose your resource.	**Layer in detail.**	**Anchor it physically**	**Breathe it in**	**Practice returning**
Recall a time, place, or person that gave you a sense of safety, calm, or strength.	Notice colors, sounds, textures, and the felt sense in your body as you bring it closer.	Place a hand on your heart, hold your wrist, or choose another grounding touch.	With each inhale, imagine your body absorbing this resource. Stay with it for 30–60 seconds.	Repeat until it becomes easier to access on demand.

SECTION FIVE

Other People's Reactions – When the World Doesn't Get It

One of the deepest wounds after miscarriage isn't always the loss itself — it's the silence that follows. The awkwardness. The quick change of subject. The well-meaning comments that land like knives. You might hear, "At least it was early," or "You can try again," or worst of all, nothing at all. The world, it seems, has a hard time holding space for grief that doesn't have a visible marker — no funeral, no photos, no timeline of "acceptable mourning."

This section is for the part of you that feels erased by how others responded — or didn't. It's for the anger, confusion, loneliness, and disconnection that can surface when people don't get it. We'll explore how to honor your grief even when others can't, how to protect your space, and how to advocate for your needs without shame. You don't owe anyone a softened version of your loss. Your pain is real — even when they don't see it.

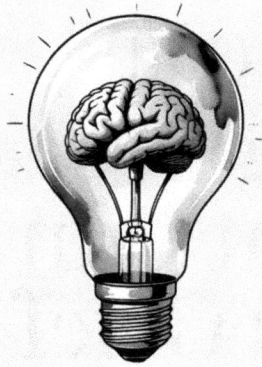

Making Sense Of It
Navigating a World That Can't Hold Your Grief

After miscarriage, one of the most jarring aspects isn't just the loss itself — it's how others respond, or fail to respond. Humans are social creatures, wired to seek attunement, validation, and acknowledgment from those around us. When your grief is minimized, deflected, or met with awkward silence, it can trigger a cascade of emotions: confusion, anger, hurt, and even a creeping sense of isolation. Your mind notices the mismatch between what you feel and what the world allows you to express, and your nervous system responds as though there is a subtle threat — not from danger, but from disconnection.

This response is deeply rooted in psychology. When humans experience loss, the brain searches for mirrors — people or rituals that reflect our pain back to us. Without these reflections, grief feels unmoored. Comments meant to console — "At least it was early," or "You can try again" — may unintentionally reinforce a sense of invisibility. Even silence, often offered out of discomfort, signals that your emotional reality is not being held. Over time, repeated invalidation can teach your nervous system that expressing grief is unsafe, prompting withdrawal, numbing, or hyper-vigilance in social situations.

Socially and culturally, miscarriage is one of the most misunderstood losses. Unlike deaths of adults or children, there are few formal rituals or expectations around mourning, leaving loved ones unsure how to respond. Some may avoid the topic entirely, while others attempt "fixes" that unintentionally diminish the significance of your loss.

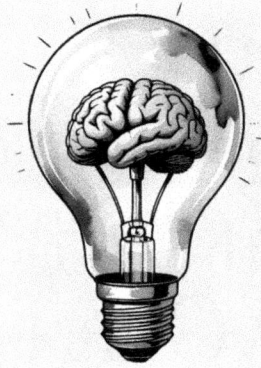

Making Sense Of It
Navigating a World That Can't Hold Your Grief

This cultural discomfort amplifies the loneliness of grief, creating a subtle pressure to minimize your feelings, act composed, or even perform resilience for the comfort of others.

Anthropological research on mourning shows that when societies lack public acknowledgment of loss, individuals often invent personal rituals or symbolic gestures to create meaning. The absence of shared recognition doesn't diminish grief — it simply requires that you create your own containers, your own mirrors. Acknowledging the mismatch between your inner world and others' responses is the first step toward regaining agency.

Psychologically, navigating others' reactions requires two things: noticing the impact of misunderstanding without internalizing blame, and reclaiming your authority over your grief. You may choose when, how, and to whom you express your emotions. You may set micro-boundaries — deciding what questions to answer, what conversations to engage in, or even when to step away. These choices are not defensive walls; they are affirmations that your grief is real, valid, and worthy of space — even when others cannot provide it.

Grieving in a world that doesn't fully get it is a quiet, ongoing negotiation. By observing the dynamics without judgment, giving yourself permission to feel unacknowledged anger or sadness, and creating your own mirrors of support.

Who did you most hope would show up for you — and how did they respond?

Let yourself be honest. Whether someone disappeared, said something hurtful, or tried but couldn't meet you emotionally, reflect on how their response impacted you and your ability to grieve fully.

Who did you most hope would show up for you — and how did they respond?

_____

_____

_____

_____

_____

_____

_____

_____

_____

_____

_____

_____

_____

_____

_____

_____

_____

_____

What has been the hardest or most painful comment someone made about your loss?

Write it down, not to relive the pain but to acknowledge what stuck with you. Then ask: Why did this hurt so much? What did I need instead?

What has been the hardest or most painful comment someone made about your loss?

Have you felt pressure to hide or minimize your miscarriage to make others comfortable?

Reflect on the moments you've swallowed your pain, smiled through it, or stayed silent. What did that cost you? What did it protect you from?

Have you felt pressure to hide or minimize your miscarriage to make others comfortable?

What would you say to someone if you were fully safe to speak your truth?

Imagine you could express your pain, anger, or disappointment without fear of judgment. Write a letter — even if you never send it — and say what your heart needs to say.

What would you say to someone if you were fully safe to speak your truth?

How have other people's reactions shaped the way you view your own grief?

Explore whether their invalidation caused you to doubt your feelings, question your right to mourn, or turn inward. What beliefs might need to be gently rewritten?

How have other people's reactions shaped the way you view your own grief?

Who has shown up for you — even in small ways?

Bring attention to the people or moments that made you feel seen. Let their care register in your nervous system. Even small kindnesses matter.

Who has shown up for you — even in small ways?

What boundaries do you wish you could set (or have already set) around this grief?

Do you need space from certain people? Limits around conversations? Permission to walk away from emotional labor? Write out what boundaries would support your healing.

What boundaries do you wish you could set (or have already set) around this grief?

TRACING THE TRUTH

REACTION RADAR

Other people's responses can feel like echoes bouncing off your grief — some supportive, some jarring, some silent. This exercise helps you map how different reactions land, giving you clarity on which connections hold you and which leave you feeling unseen.

Why it helps:
Visualizing responses allows you to step back from emotional overwhelm and see relational patterns. It highlights which connections nurture your grief and which may need boundaries or intentional distance.

Draw a circle in the center of a page labeled Me & My Grief.
Around that circle, write the names of people you've shared your loss with, or who have witnessed your grief indirectly.
Next to each name, note the type of reaction you received: silence, well-meaning advice, awkwardness, avoidance, or support.
Use symbols or colors to mark how each response made you feel: hurt, invalidated, comforted, frustrated, or unseen.

Reflect on patterns: Which reactions helped you feel held? Which amplified isolation? Which triggered anger or self-doubt?

TRACING THE TRUTH

REACTION RADAR

TRACING THE TRUTH

MY NEEDS SCRIPT

It's easy to feel silenced or overlooked when others don't understand your loss. This exercise helps you define what you need and how to ask for it, giving your grief a voice without apology or compromise.

Why it helps:
Misunderstanding can leave grief feeling invisible. This exercise transforms feelings of frustration into actionable statements, empowering you to reclaim agency over how your loss is witnessed and respected.

In What I Need, write specific support you wish others could offer — listening without advice, space to grieve, or acknowledgement of your loss.
In How I Can Express It, write down simple phrases you could use: e.g., "I appreciate you caring, but I need to process this on my own for now," or "I need you to just listen without giving advice."

Practice saying these aloud or in your mind to build confidence and internalize permission to protect your emotional space.

TRACING THE TRUTH

MY NEEDS SCRIPT

What I Need	How I Can Express It

WORRY WINDOW

Worries often hijack your mind, showing up at every unexpected moment. By giving them a dedicated "time slot," you reclaim control instead of letting them run your day. This practice teaches your nervous system that there's a safe space and a safe time to process, so you're not constantly reacting to every intrusive thought. During the window, you can gently evaluate what's actionable versus what you need to let go, building clarity and self-trust. Outside the window, a simple cue like "not now—later" helps you return to the present without guilt or shame. Over time, this simple structure reduces the intensity and frequency of anxious loops.

Park your worries: Write them down as they arise.

....

....

....

....

....

Set a 15-minute window: Choose a consistent time each day for processing.

_____

Outside the window: Use a cue phrase like "not now—later" to return to your day.

Inside the window: Review the list. Solve what's actionable, accept what isn't, and release judgment.

Close the window: End with a grounding or soothing activity to signal completion.

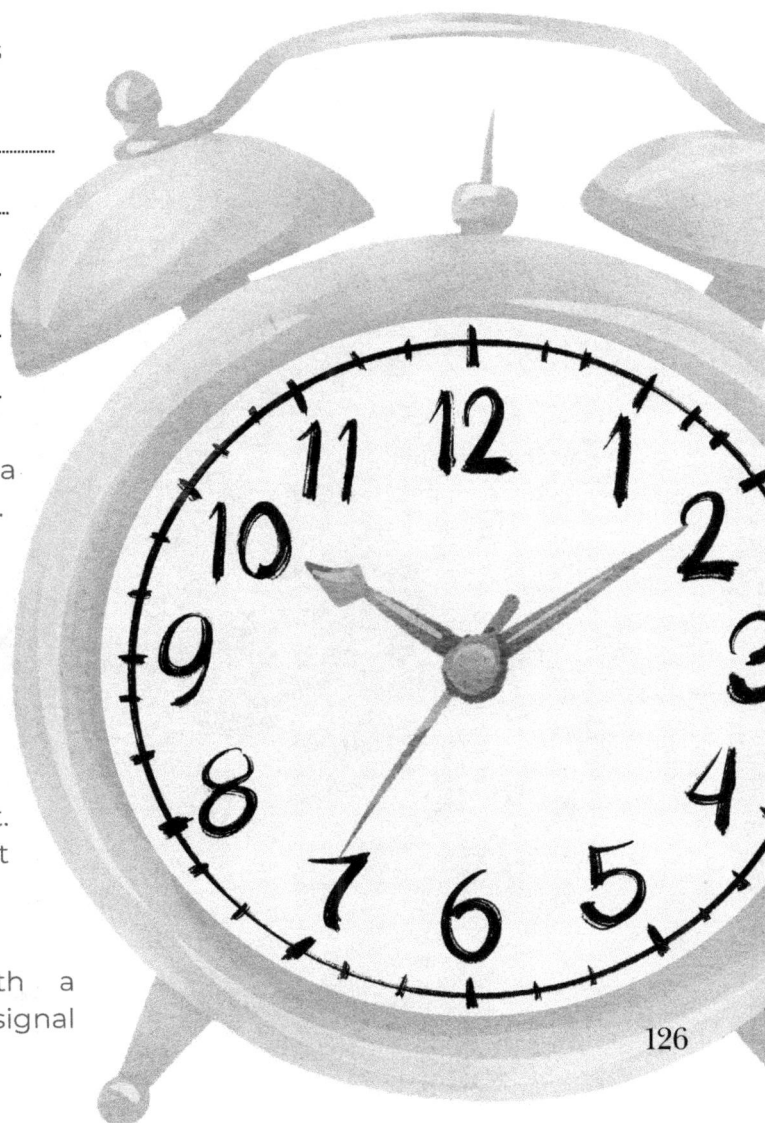

GENTLE BREATH FOCUS

When anxiety spikes, the mind and body race together — thoughts accelerate, heart rate climbs, muscles tighten. Counting your breath gives both something steady to follow. By pairing inhale and exhale with numbers, you create a gentle anchor that slows the nervous system, refocuses attention, and interrupts spiraling thoughts. This isn't about perfection or achieving ten — it's about returning to the rhythm whenever distraction occurs. Even a few minutes daily strengthens your capacity to notice tension, settle your body, and move through anxious moments with less overwhelm.

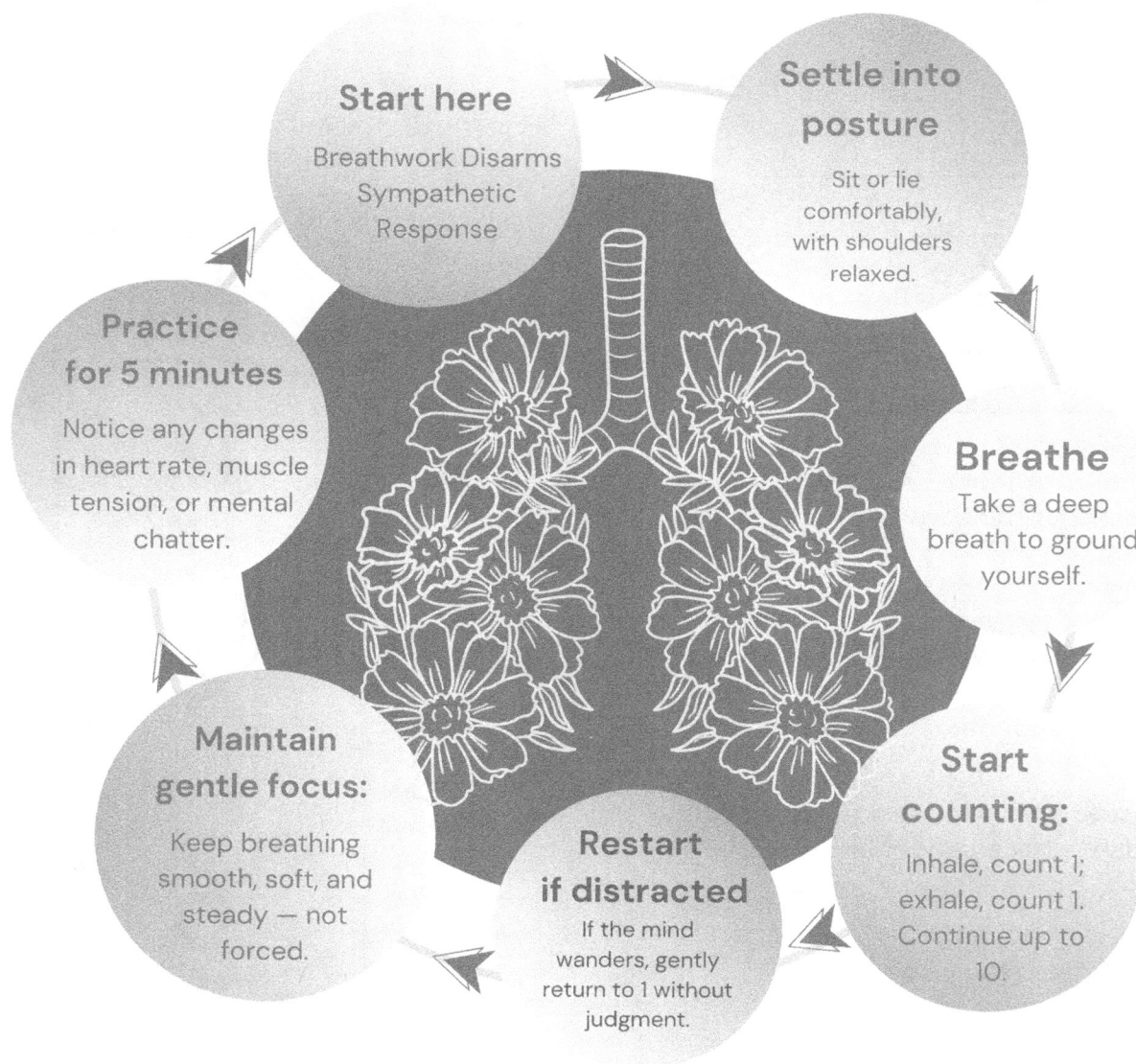

Start here
Breathwork Disarms Sympathetic Response

Settle into posture
Sit or lie comfortably, with shoulders relaxed.

Breathe
Take a deep breath to ground yourself.

Start counting:
Inhale, count 1; exhale, count 1. Continue up to 10.

Restart if distracted
If the mind wanders, gently return to 1 without judgment.

Maintain gentle focus:
Keep breathing smooth, soft, and steady — not forced.

Practice for 5 minutes
Notice any changes in heart rate, muscle tension, or mental chatter.

FEAR SCALE

Anxiety loves to inflate danger — suddenly a minor stressor feels like the end of the world. The Catastrophe Scale helps you step back and see the actual size of the threat. By putting a number on it and comparing it to your personal "0–100" life scale, you can measure proportion instead of panic. This clarifies what truly deserves energy and what doesn't, allowing your nervous system to respond appropriately rather than overreact. Over time, practicing this recalibration reduces automatic catastrophizing and builds confidence in your ability to face fears without being hijacked by them.

Identify the feared event and imagine it fully.

Rate it: Place it on a 0–100 scale where 0 is no impact and 100 is a true catastrophe.

Check extremes: Ask yourself, "What would a 90 look like? A 10?" to anchor your scale.

Place the fear: Decide the most accurate number for this specific event.

Choose a proportionate response: Match your actions and energy to the real size of the event.

SECTION SIX

Pregnancy After Loss – Hope, Fear, and Not Trusting the Joy Yet

If you're pregnant again after a miscarriage, you may be living in a strange, quiet tug-of-war between hope and dread. People might congratulate you, expecting you to smile, glow, and celebrate. But inside, you might be waiting for the floor to fall out again. Every cramp, every quiet moment might send your body into panic. You may find yourself scrolling for symptoms, holding your breath during ultrasounds, or feeling numb when you wish you could feel joy.

This section is for you if you're walking through a new pregnancy with your guard still up — not because you're ungrateful, but because your body remembers what it's like to lose. We'll explore what it means to hold space for both fear and hope, how to soften into this moment without betraying the past, and how to connect with this pregnancy in your own time, on your own terms. You are not failing at joy. You are protecting your heart.

130

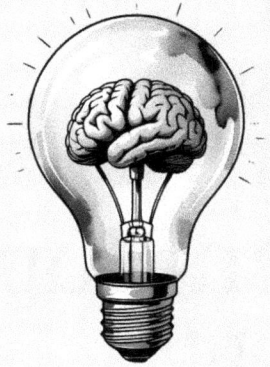

Making Sense Of It
The Nervous System Between Hope and Fear

Pregnancy after loss is unlike any other experience. Your body and mind carry memory — not just of physical miscarriage, but of the trauma encoded in your nervous system. Neuroscience shows that the brain doesn't differentiate fully between past trauma and current potential threat; your nervous system remembers what it felt like to lose, and it reacts as though danger is still present. This is why even a fleeting cramp, a quiet moment, or a routine ultrasound can trigger heightened alertness, anxiety, or emotional shutdown. Your mind may be whispering, Be careful, don't get attached, while your heart simultaneously longs to believe in this life.

This tension between hope and fear is not a failure. It is a survival response, rooted in a system designed to protect you from harm. Psychologists call this anticipatory grief — the mourning of potential loss even while holding a fragile thread of joy. It's a paradox: your heart wants to feel, but your nervous system wants to survive. Understanding this paradox can be profoundly freeing. When you recognize that fear is biologically anchored, you begin to give yourself permission to inhabit both hope and anxiety without judgment.

Sociologically, there is also immense pressure to display "normal" excitement. Society expects glowing announcements, smiling ultrasound photos, and visible celebrations.

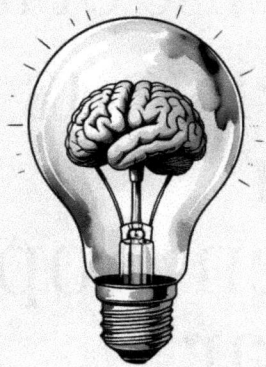

Making Sense Of It
The Nervous System Between Hope and Fear

For someone carrying past trauma, these expectations can create an additional layer of guilt: guilt for not feeling joy fully, guilt for protecting your emotions, guilt for needing space. These pressures are external mirrors that can amplify internal tension, making you question whether you are "doing it right."

Embodiment is central here. Trauma is stored in the body: shallow breath, tight shoulders, clenched jaw, racing heart. Mindfulness, breath awareness, and somatic exercises are not just soothing — they are essential tools to reconnect with safety signals, allowing you to inhabit your body without being hijacked by past loss. The body remembers loss, but it can also relearn safety, trust, and grounded joy when given care and attunement.

The transformative insight is this: your fear and hope are not opposing forces — they are coexisting truths. Protecting your heart does not betray your joy; acknowledging anxiety does not block love. By observing your nervous system, naming your anticipatory grief, and giving yourself permission to feel ambivalence, you reclaim agency over a process that can feel entirely unpredictable. You are not failing at joy — you are surviving, attuning, and learning to carry hope alongside fear in a way that honors both the past and this new life.

What emotions have come up during this pregnancy that surprised you?

Let yourself name what's been confusing, scary, or different from what you expected — even if it's anger, guilt, or numbness.

What emotions have come up during this pregnancy that surprised you?

In what moments do you feel most afraid — and what do those moments remind you of?

Fear often carries memory. Explore what past losses your current anxiety may be echoing.

In what moments do you feel most afraid — and what do those
moments remind you of?

What parts of you are trying to protect you right now?

Identify the voices that say, "Don't get too excited," or "This might not last." What are they afraid of? What do they need?

What parts of you are trying to protect you right now?

Have you felt pressure to be "positive" about this pregnancy — and how has that affected you?

Reflect on whether others' expectations have made you feel like your fears or grief aren't allowed. What would it feel like to be fully honest?

Have you felt pressure to be "positive" about this pregnancy — and how has that affected you?

How can you let yourself connect with this pregnancy without demanding certainty?

Explore gentle ways to bond or acknowledge this new life — even if it's just in quiet, private moments.

How can you let yourself connect with this pregnancy without demanding certainty?

What would it look like to grieve and hope at the same time?

Can you allow both parts of you — the one who remembers the loss, and the one who wants to believe again — to coexist?

LESSONS IN INK

After hardship, the brain often circles around the why — why it happened, why you stayed, why you're still hurting. Meaning-making is a way to gently reclaim authorship. By naming what you survived and drawing out what it taught you about your own values and limits, you shift from being swallowed by the story to becoming the narrator of it. This process isn't about silver linings or forced positivity. It's about grounding your pain in context — saying, this mattered, this shaped me, and here's what I'm carrying forward. Closing with a boundary sets a line in the sand: you're not just reflecting on what happened, you're deciding how it changes the way you'll protect yourself in the future.

Headline: Write a short, bold line that sums up what you survived (as if it were on the front page of your personal newspaper).

Lessons: List 3–5 things it revealed about your needs, your limits, or your values.

Boundary: Write one clear, non-negotiable boundary you'll honor from now on.

HOLDING HARD DATES

When difficult anniversaries come around—whether it's the day everything fell apart, a loss, or a traumatic turning point—the body remembers even when the mind tries not to. This can show up as anxiety, fatigue, irritability, or old grief bubbling back. Creating an intentional ritual allows you to meet those days with structure instead of being blindsided. By noting the date ahead of time, building in gentle scaffolding (like a support person, a nourishing activity, and less demand on yourself), you create a container for your nervous system. Closing the day with gratitude is not about being thankful for the pain itself, but for your endurance—that you lived through it, and you're still here. Ritual turns an overwhelming anniversary into a moment of honoring resilience.

Mark the Date
Note the anniversary on your calendar so it doesn't sneak up.

Plan Support
Choose one person you can reach out to if things feel heavy.

Nourish
Schedule at least one grounding or soothing activity (walk, bath, journaling, cozy meal).

Lighten the Load
Keep your to-do list small that day.

Close with Gratitude
End the evening by writing or saying one thing you're grateful for in your survival.

146

SECTION SEVEN

Already a Parent – Making Space for Grief When You Have to Keep Going

Grieving a miscarriage while parenting other children can feel like living in two separate worlds. One part of you is broken, quiet, and aching. The other part must stay awake, feed snacks, manage tantrums, show up for bedtime, and keep the world spinning for little ones who may never know what you lost. You might feel pulled in opposite directions — guilty for grieving, guilty for smiling, guilty for not "being enough" in either space.

This section is here to hold the truth of that impossible in-between. You are not doing it wrong. You are a human navigating real, complicated emotions while still being needed by others. That's not weakness — that's endurance. We'll explore how to create moments of inner space for grief, how to talk about loss with children (if you choose to), and how to tend to your own heart while still parenting the ones in front of you. You deserve care too.

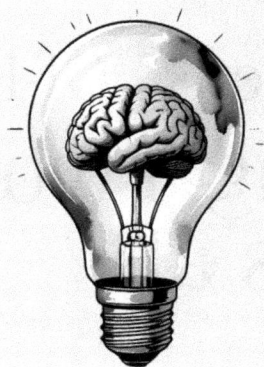

Making Sense Of It
Holding Two Worlds at Once

Grieving a miscarriage while caring for living children creates a tension that is both invisible and relentless. Psychologically, this experience engages what researchers call role conflict — the simultaneous demands of two identities that can feel incompatible. One part of you is engulfed in grief, mourning what could have been. The other must show up, perform, and provide for children who rely on you. Both are real, valid, and non-negotiable parts of your life, yet the push and pull can feel exhausting and isolating.

Neuroscience offers insight into why this tension can feel so physically taxing. Grief triggers the body's stress response: heightened cortisol, muscle tension, shallow breathing, and disrupted sleep. Parenting, especially in active or demanding moments, requires executive function, emotional regulation, and energy reserves. When grief and caregiving collide, your nervous system is essentially multitasking between survival mode and caregiving mode, leaving little room for internal processing. This is why fatigue, irritability, and emotional fragmentation are so common — your body and brain are constantly negotiating two high-stakes realities at once.

Social and cultural pressures exacerbate this tension. Parents are expected to be resilient, cheerful, and fully available to their children, while grief is often treated as private, invisible, or inconvenient. These unspoken expectations can create guilt loops: guilt for crying in secret, guilt for being joyful with your living children, guilt for wishing for the child you lost.

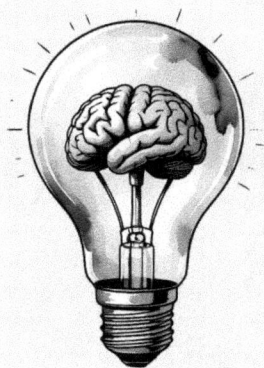

Making Sense Of It
Holding Two Worlds at Once

It is not weakness to feel conflicted — it is the natural response of a human mind and body stretched across simultaneous, urgent demands.

Understanding this dynamic allows you to reclaim agency and self-compassion. Structuring moments of intentional presence with grief — even five quiet minutes to journal, breathe, or hold a symbolic ritual — signals to your nervous system that mourning is safe, even in the middle of life's chaos. Similarly, when interacting with children, acknowledging your capacity limits and using mindful parenting techniques allows you to be present without erasing your own needs. You can model emotional resilience without needing to suppress grief, showing children that complexity, sorrow, and love can coexist.

The transformative insight here is that these dual realities are not in conflict — they are coexisting layers of human experience. By observing the tension without judgment, giving yourself permission to feel fully, and carving intentional spaces for grief, you nurture both your own heart and the children in your care. Endurance does not require perfection; it requires acknowledgment, compassion, and the courage to hold both worlds without sacrificing either.

Where in your day does your grief go when you're parenting?

Does it get pushed aside? Show up in your body? Leak out as irritation or numbness? Give it some gentle attention.

Where in your day does your grief go when you're parenting?

What would your grief say if it could speak freely, without worrying about your children hearing?

Write a letter from your grief, no filter, no judgment. Let it speak its whole truth.

What would your grief say if it could speak freely, without worrying about your children hearing?

What parts of you feel pressure to "stay strong," and what are they afraid might happen if you fall apart?

Explore the protective roles you play, and what those parts need in return.

What parts of you feel pressure to "stay strong," and what are they afraid might happen if you fall apart?

When do you feel most connected to your children right now? When do you feel farthest away?

Without blame, notice the rhythms. This can help you stay anchored in your own truth.

When do you feel most connected to your children right now?
When do you feel farthest away?

What kind of support would allow you to grieve without guilt?

Imagine practical, emotional, or spiritual support — even if it feels far away right now.

_____

_____

_____

_____

_____

_____

_____

_____

_____

_____

_____

_____

What kind of support would allow you to grieve without guilt?

How can you create small rituals of connection — for both the child you lost and the children you're raising?

Explore gentle, simple ways to acknowledge both bonds without overextending yourself.

How can you create small rituals of connection — for both the child you lost and the children you're raising?

TRACING THE TRUTH

TALKING ABOUT THE BABY WITH CHILDREN

Children are sensitive to loss, even when it isn't physically visible, and they may sense your sadness before you speak. This exercise is designed to help you communicate gently and honestly, in age-appropriate ways, without placing blame or creating confusion. It's not about giving them all the answers — it's about acknowledging the loss and reassuring them.

Why it helps:
This exercise helps children understand loss without fear or self-blame, and gives parents a structured way to communicate while still processing their own grief. It honors both your emotional reality and your child's need for safety and clarity.

Use clear, simple words: Keep explanations concrete, brief, and age-appropriate.
Example: "The baby in my belly stopped growing. We're very sad. It's not your fault."

Name your feelings: Modeling emotional expression teaches children that it's safe to feel.
Example: "I feel really sad sometimes. You might see me cry. That's okay. Crying helps."

Invite their feelings: Allow space for curiosity, confusion, or uncertainty.
Example: "Do you have any questions? It's okay to feel sad, or confused, or not know what to say."

Create a gentle ritual (if desired): Rituals help children (and you) externalize and process grief.
Light a candle, draw a picture, plant a flower — something symbolic that acknowledges the loss.

Reassure their safety: Safety and love are the anchor for children, even in moments of shared grief.
Example: "I love you. We're going to be okay. Even when I'm sad, I'm still your parent."

PROGRESSIVE MUSCLE RELAXATION

When stress lingers, tension builds in muscles without us noticing, keeping the nervous system on high alert. PMR gently signals to your body that it's safe to let go. By intentionally tensing and then releasing each muscle group, you highlight the difference between tension and relaxation, training your body to notice and release stress. This practice doesn't just relax the muscles—it communicates to your nervous system that it can downshift, making calm feel real and accessible.

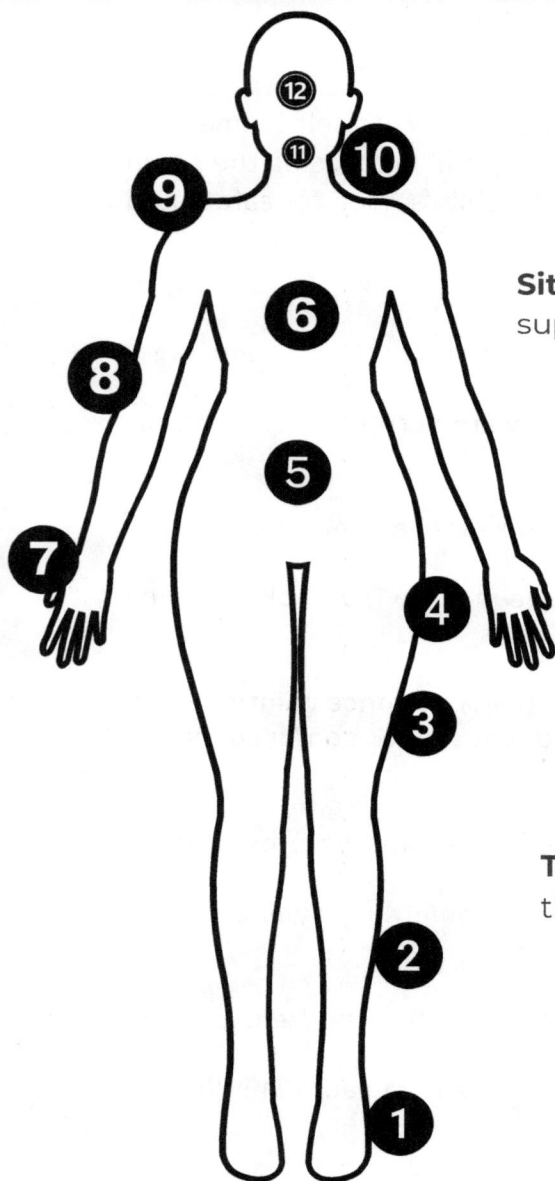

Sit or lie comfortably with your body supported.

Starting at your feet, tense the muscles for 3–5 seconds, then exhale and release.

Move upward through calves, thighs, glutes, stomach, back, hands, arms, shoulders, neck, jaw, face, tensing and releasing each group.

As you release, imagine tension melting away or flowing out of your body.

Take a few normal breaths and notice the overall sense of ease.

165

THE VOO RESET

Our vagus nerve connects the brain and body, regulating stress and calm. Gentle vocalization, like a long "voo" on the exhale, stimulates this pathway, sending a signal that it's safe to downshift arousal. The vibration through your chest and throat also grounds your attention in your body, giving your nervous system tangible proof that it can relax. Just a few rounds can reduce tension, slow your heart rate, and invite a sense of ease.

Sit or stand comfortably with shoulders relaxed.

Inhale slowly through your nose.

Exhale while vocalizing a long, gentle "voo," letting your chest and throat vibrate.

Repeat for 3 rounds, noticing the sensations and any shift in tension.

Place a hand on your chest to feel the vibration more clearly.

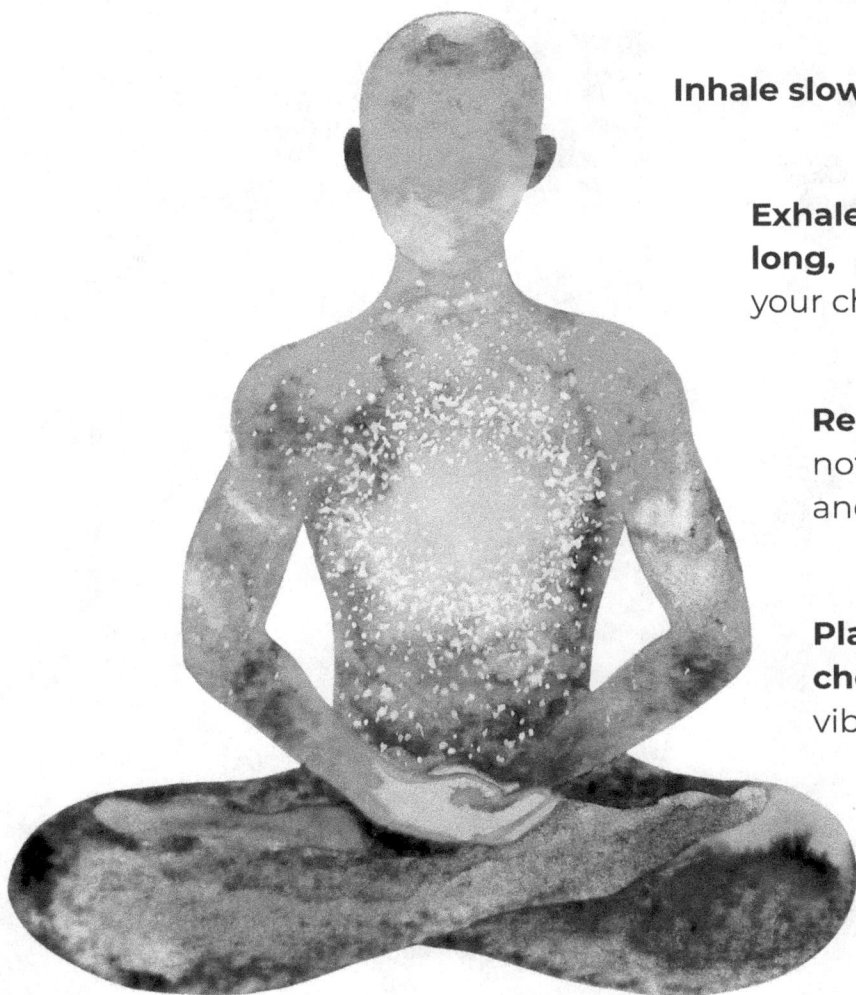

SECTION EIGHT

When Family Doesn't Understand – Dealing with Dismissive, Hurtful, or Silent Reactions

One of the deepest wounds in miscarriage grief can come not from the loss itself, but from the reactions — or absence of them — from the people you expected to show up. The family member who changes the subject. The one who says, "At least it was early." The silence from those who never even acknowledged it happened. These moments can make your grief feel not just invisible, but invalidated — as if you're being asked to mourn quietly so no one else has to be uncomfortable.

This section is here to help you reclaim the truth of your experience, even when others can't or won't reflect it back. You'll learn how to set boundaries with compassion, how to protect your story from people who can't hold it, and how to let yourself grieve without waiting for others to catch up. You are allowed to need more. You are allowed to name the pain of being unseen.

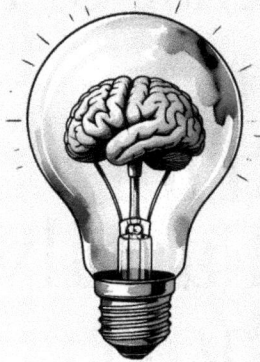

Making Sense Of It
Reclaiming Your Grief When Family Falls Short

Grief is social by nature. From birth onward, humans are wired to seek acknowledgment, attunement, and reflection from those closest to us — especially family. When miscarriage occurs, the expectation is that loved ones will witness, support, and hold space for your sorrow. When they fail to do so, whether through dismissal, avoidance, or silence, it can feel profoundly isolating. Psychologists refer to this as disenfranchised grief, a type of loss that society, and even your closest relationships, fail to validate. What makes it particularly painful with family is the added layer of relational history: the people who fail to see you are often the very ones whose recognition matters most.

Neuroscience explains why these reactions feel like more than disappointment. When your emotional experience is minimized, your nervous system interprets the lack of acknowledgment as a social threat. Cortisol rises, the body tenses, and hyper-vigilance can emerge — a quiet alert that says: I cannot rely on these people to hold my emotional reality. Over time, repeated dismissals can even create patterns of self-doubt, making you question whether your grief is valid or whether you are "overreacting."

Family responses are shaped by culture, personal experience, and discomfort with reproductive loss. Many relatives respond with silence or clichés because they themselves are anxious, unequipped, or constrained by societal norms that treat miscarriage as private, invisible, or inconvenient.

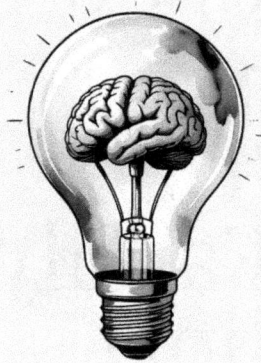

Making Sense Of It
Reclaiming Your Grief When Family Falls Short

Understanding this does not erase the pain, but it can shift your focus: the problem lies not in your grief, but in the inability of others to meet it.

Reclaiming agency in this context involves three key strategies: recognition, boundary-setting, and self-validation. First, name your emotions clearly and acknowledge the ways family reactions impact you. Second, define what you need — space, selective sharing, or limiting contact — and communicate boundaries with compassion but firmness. Third, cultivate internal attunement: when family cannot reflect your grief, you reflect it back to yourself. Journaling, ritual, or private acknowledgment creates a container for your loss, sending a powerful message to your nervous system that your emotions are legitimate.

Transformative insight comes in realizing that validation does not need to come from others to be true. Your grief is real, worthy, and deserving of attention. Even when family cannot hold it, you can create safe spaces for your emotions, honor the depth of your loss, and protect your heart from further invalidation. In doing so, you step fully into your experience, claim your story, and demonstrate that being unseen by others does not make you invisible — it makes your grief your own.

Whose response to your miscarriage has hurt the most, and why?

Try to name the moment and what you needed that you didn't receive.

Whose response to your miscarriage has hurt the most, and why?

What part of you feels silenced or invisible around certain people?

Explore how this part tries to protect you and what it wishes others could understand.

What part of you feels silenced or invisible around certain people?

What have you tried to tell others about your grief — and how have they responded?

Reflect on what felt helpful or harmful. This can guide future boundaries.

What have you tried to tell others about your grief — and how have they responded?

What messages (spoken or unspoken) have you received from family about how grief "should" look?

Are any of these messages outdated, harmful, or ready to be challenged?

What messages (spoken or unspoken) have you received from family about how grief "should" look?

If you could hear the perfect validating words from someone right now, what would they be?

Write them out — even if you have to say them to yourself.

If you could hear the perfect validating words from someone right now, what would they be?

Where do you still feel pressure to "move on," and what does that pressure cost you?

Let yourself be honest. You're allowed to take your time.

Where do you still feel pressure to "move on," and what does that pressure cost you?

TRACING THE TRUTH

MAPPING FAMILY RESPONSES

Family can be both a source of support and, at times, misunderstanding. This exercise helps you see, without judgment, how each family member responds to your grief. By mapping reactions, you gain clarity on patterns and where you may need emotional space.

Why it helps:
Visualizing responses removes emotional overwhelm and highlights relational patterns. It allows you to understand where support exists, where you may need distance, and empowers you to make conscious choices about engagement.

Draw a simple diagram: a circle in the center labeled Me & My Grief.
Around the circle, write the names of family members you've shared your loss with (or who are aware).
Next to each name, note their typical responses: supportive, dismissive, silent, well-meaning but awkward, or other.
Use symbols or colors to indicate how each response affects you emotionally: comforted, frustrated, unseen, anxious, or validated.

Reflect: Which relationships nurture your grief? Which amplify pain? Are there boundaries you need to protect your emotional space?

TRACING THE TRUTH

MAPPING FAMILY RESPONSES

PROTECTIVE BUBBLE

When emotions run high or interactions feel draining, it's easy for your energy to get scattered. Imagining a soft, light bubble around you helps create a sense of personal space and safety. Using your breath to strengthen the bubble on the inhale and filter in only what feels nourishing on the exhale trains your nervous system to notice boundaries, giving you a calm, centered feeling even in challenging situations.

Sit or stand comfortably, spine tall.

Visualize a soft bubble surrounding your body, glowing lightly.

Inhale and imagine the bubble strengthening, expanding slightly.

Exhale and let in only what nourishes — warmth, safety, or calm.

Continue for 1–3 minutes, noticing a sense of energetic protection and centeredness.

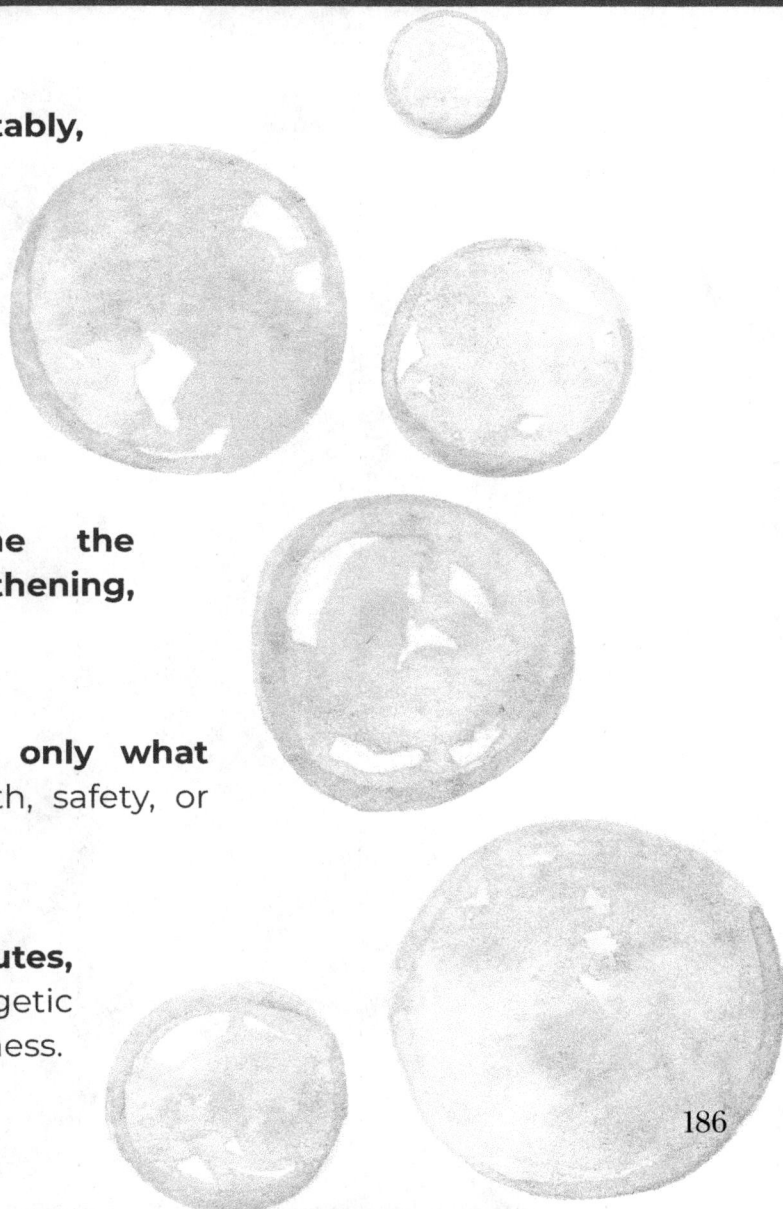

SOFT EYES RESET

When we're anxious or hypervigilant, our gaze often narrows, making the world feel tense or threatening. Softening your eyes and expanding your peripheral vision sends a signal to your nervous system that it's safe to relax. This subtle shift can reduce tension in the shoulders, jaw, and chest, helping you feel steadier and more grounded, even in moments of stress.

Sit or stand comfortably with spine tall.

Focus softly ahead, allowing your peripheral vision to widen.

Notice objects to the sides without staring directly at them.

Pay attention to how your body responds — shoulders, jaw, and breath may soften naturally.

Continue for 1–2 minutes, gently returning your focus to soft vision whenever it narrows.

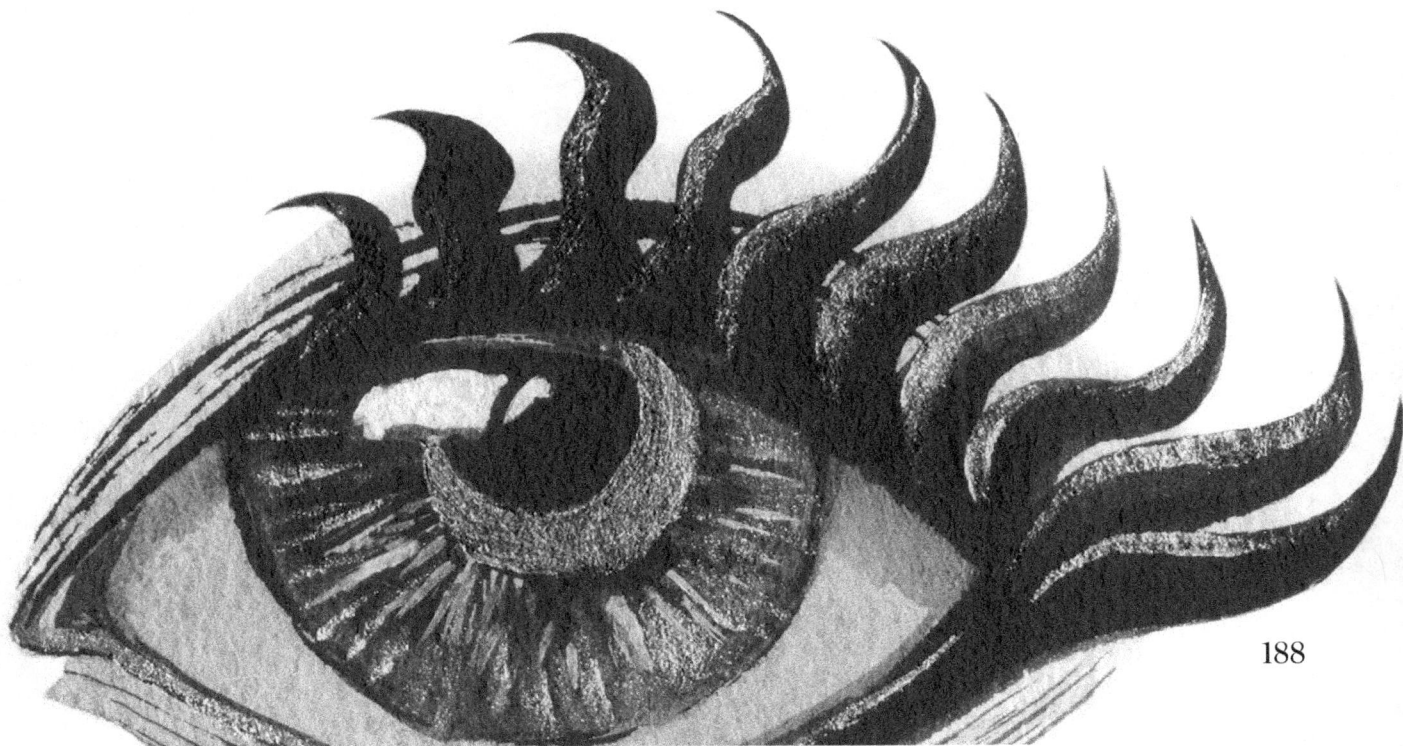

SECTION NINE

The World Moves On – But I'm Still Not Okay

There's a strange loneliness that settles in after the cards stop coming, the check-ins dwindle, and the world expects you to be "back to normal." Grief doesn't follow a polite schedule, but life around you seems to — coworkers expect your focus, friends expect your presence, and even loved ones may start to grow silent. Inside, you may still feel like the world has shattered. Outside, it seems like it never paused at all.

This section is for the quiet, aching space between visible crisis and invisible grief — where the support has faded, but your pain hasn't. It's not that you're ungrateful for the people who tried to be there. It's just that their timeline doesn't match your reality. Here, we'll talk about navigating life when others seem ready for you to move on — but you're still right in the middle of it. Because your grief is not behind you. It's still here. And that's okay.

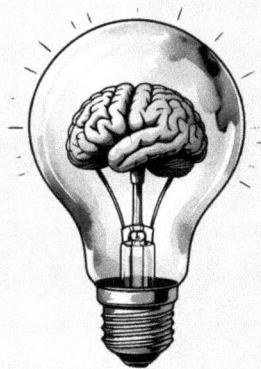

Making Sense Of It
The Gap Between Inner Grief and Outer Expectation

One of the most painful aspects of miscarriage is the widening gap between what's happening inside you and how the world responds. Inside, you may feel raw, shattered, or suspended in time — heart aching, thoughts spinning, body carrying tension you can't release. Outside, the world moves on. Friends stop asking. Colleagues expect productivity. Even loved ones seem to glance away, unsure how to hold your pain. That mismatch creates a kind of emotional dissonance, as though you're being asked to perform healing you haven't yet felt.

Psychologically, this is a rupture between internal reality — your emotions, thoughts, and bodily sensations — and external reality, the feedback, silence, or expectations from others. When grief is invisible or minimized, self-doubt can creep in. Am I overreacting? Am I stuck? Am I failing? This is grief invalidation, and it's profoundly common after miscarriage because there's no social ritual, public acknowledgment, or clear timeline to mark what you've lost. The grief is real, but society often fails to recognize it in ways that allow mourning to be fully witnessed.

The Dual Process Model of grief illuminates why this is so destabilizing. Healthy mourning requires oscillation: moving between loss-oriented tasks (facing your grief, remembering, crying, honoring what's lost) and restoration-oriented tasks (managing daily responsibilities, caring for others, returning to routine).

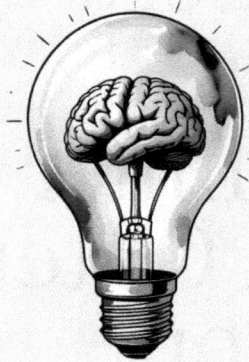

Making Sense Of It
The Gap Between Inner Grief and Outer Expectation

But when the external world signals, Move on, smile, keep going, this rhythm is interrupted. You may find yourself emotionally stuck — not because you're failing at healing, but because the world hasn't given your grief the space it needs to breathe.

This dissonance can ripple into body and mind: emotional numbness, anxiety, intrusive thoughts, shame, and self-silencing become common strategies to navigate a world that doesn't pause for your loss. You might smile when inside you ache, push down tears to function, or hide your grief to avoid awkwardness. Over time, this can burden your nervous system, fracture your sense of connection, and slow the natural healing process.

The transformative insight is that your grief remains valid, even when unseen. The external world does not set the timeline for your healing. By acknowledging the gap, naming it, and creating intentional spaces to feel, remember, and honor your loss, you reclaim agency over your mourning. You allow your inner reality to exist fully, even in a world that has moved on, and begin to bridge the distance between what you feel and how you live.

What has the world expected from me that I haven't been ready to give?

Explore how others' timelines have made you feel — pressured, misunderstood, invisible — and what your pace truly looks like.

What has the world expected from me that I haven't been ready to give?

Where in my life have I felt most unseen in my grief?

Write about the people, spaces, or situations that didn't recognize your pain — and why that hurts.

Where in my life have I felt most unseen in my grief?

What parts of my grief feel most misunderstood — even by those closest to me?

Let yourself name the subtle, private sorrows that go unnoticed.

What parts of my grief feel most misunderstood — even by those closest to me?

What do I wish someone would say to me right now?

Give voice to the words you've needed — even if no one's spoken them.

What do I wish someone would say to me right now?

Have I started pretending to be 'fine' when I'm not? What does that cost me?

Explore the emotional toll of masking and the moments where you longed to be real.

Have I started pretending to be 'fine' when I'm not? What does that cost me?

What would it look like to stay loyal to my truth — even if others are moving on?

Imagine what it would mean to honor your timeline unapologetically.

What would it look like to stay loyal to my truth — even if others are moving on?

LEAVES ON A STREAM

We often get stuck in our thoughts, treating them as commands or facts, which fuels stress and emotional overwhelm. Defusion teaches you to step back and see thoughts as just thoughts—mental events that come and go. By visualizing them on leaves drifting down a stream, you give your mind space to notice them without reacting. This practice reduces the pull of negative thinking, strengthens present-moment awareness, and improves emotional flexibility.

Sit quietly and settle. Take a few slow breaths, noticing your body and surroundings.

Visualize the stream. Picture a gentle stream flowing in front of you.

Place thoughts on leaves. Each time a thought appears, imagine putting it on a leaf floating by.

Label hooked moments. If you notice you're caught up in a thought, gently label it "thinking" and return it to the stream.

Continue for 5–10 minutes. Keep observing without judgment, letting each thought drift away.

MOMENT-TO-MOMENT AWARENESS

Our minds are constantly busy—hearing, thinking, planning, feeling—and it's easy to get swept away in the stream of thoughts and sensations. This practice helps you step back and notice what's happening in the present without getting stuck. By softly labeling each experience, you create a gentle separation between yourself and the flood of mental activity. Even a short daily practice trains your attention, lowers emotional reactivity, and strengthens the ability to return to calm focus when life gets overwhelming.

Set a timer for 5 minutes so you can fully commit without checking the clock.

Sit comfortably and close your eyes if you like.

Notice experiences as they arise. Softly label them as: "hearing... thinking... planning... feeling..."

Return to your breath. After labeling, bring your attention back to your natural breathing.

Repeat gently. Whenever your mind wanders, notice it, label it, and return to the breath without judgment.

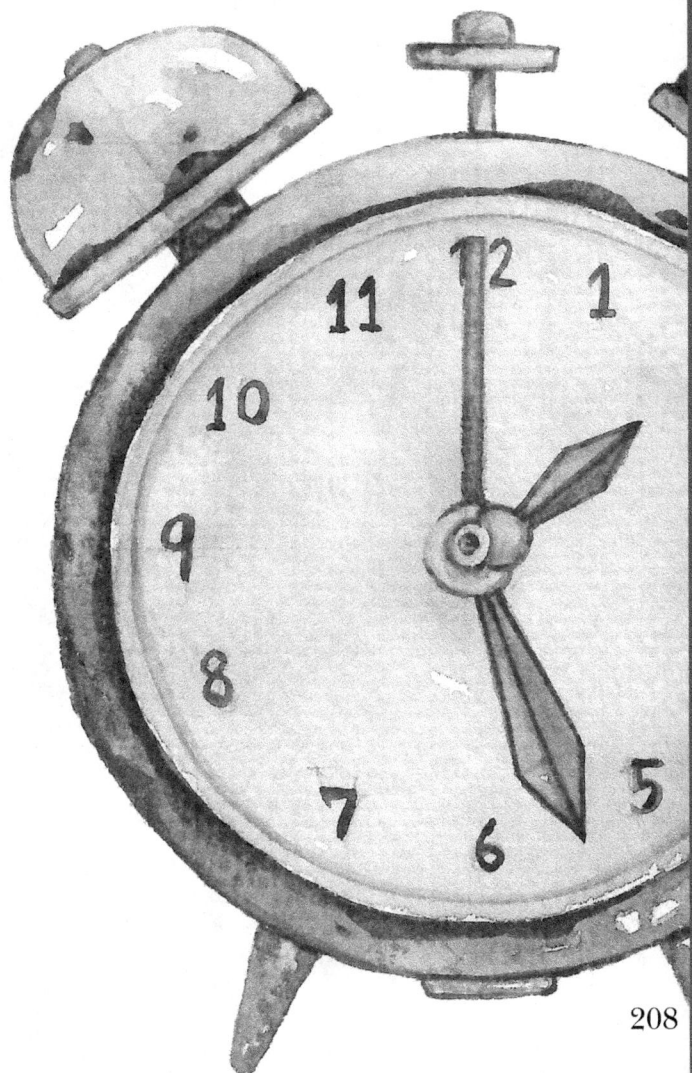

SECTION TEN

Shadows and Shame – When Grief Feels Like Failure

Miscarriage doesn't just leave behind sadness — for many, it also leaves shame. A quiet, aching sense of having failed. Failed your body. Failed your baby. Failed to do what others seem to do so easily. These thoughts are cruel, but they're common — and they often live in silence, unspoken even to those closest to us. This section is here to say: It wasn't your fault. But also, we know that hearing those words may not be enough to make them feel true. That's okay. Shame isn't logical — it's emotional. It speaks in whispers and echoes, often rooted in old wounds or impossible expectations. Whether you blame your body, your timing, your choices, or something else — this is where we begin to meet those beliefs with gentleness instead of judgment. There is nothing shameful about your grief. There is nothing shameful about your body. You did not fail. Let's begin to untangle the pain from the lie.

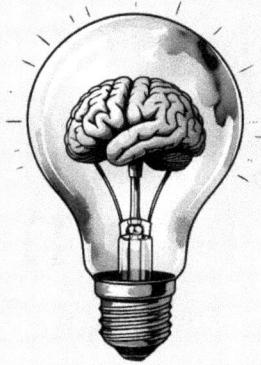

Making Sense Of It
Untangling Shame From Loss

Shame after miscarriage is often invisible, quiet, and deeply personal. Unlike grief, which can be expressed through tears, rituals, or talking, shame tends to live in silence. It whispers: You failed. You didn't do enough. You weren't enough. These thoughts may feel uniquely yours, but research shows that internalized shame after pregnancy loss is incredibly common, shaped by cultural narratives, family expectations, and personal beliefs about motherhood, timing, and bodily ability.

Psychologically, shame is an emotion rooted in self-evaluation. It signals that something about the self — not just an action or outcome — is inadequate. After miscarriage, this emotion can latch onto multiple dimensions of identity: your body, your decisions, your capacity to carry life, and even your sense of moral worth. Shame is deceptive because it feels like truth, but it is a lens, not reality. It distorts the narrative, often overlaying grief with self-criticism, and can amplify isolation as you feel "less than" or undeserving of care and support.

Socially and culturally, miscarriage often occupies an invisible space. There is little acknowledgment in public rituals or shared mourning. Combined with persistent societal messaging that women's value is tied to fertility or the ability to parent, this invisibility fuels the internal voice of failure. You may find yourself comparing your grief, your resilience, or your body's performance to others, and feeling that you fall short — even when logically, you know this is unfair.

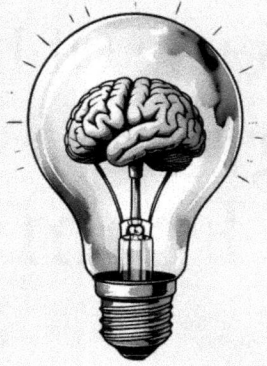

Making Sense Of It
Untangling Shame From Loss

Neuroscience shows that shame is processed in both the emotional and social regions of the brain. It triggers heightened self-consciousness, rumination, and even social withdrawal. When left unchecked, shame can reinforce negative self-beliefs and compound grief, making emotional processing heavier and more complicated.

The transformative insight is that shame is not a reflection of reality — it is a signal pointing to where your mind and heart need care, compassion, and truth. Naming it, externalizing it, and observing it without judgment are acts of radical self-compassion. You can distinguish between what truly happened (the miscarriage) and the false narratives your shame constructs. By gently challenging the messages of inadequacy, you begin to separate grief from perceived failure, creating space for honesty, self-acceptance, and healing.

Ultimately, you are not broken. You did not fail. Your grief is valid, your body is trustworthy, and your worth exists independently of outcomes, timelines, or societal expectations. Meeting shame with gentleness allows the heart to soften, the mind to witness reality, and your grief to unfold without the weight of false blame.

What are the unspoken messages I've absorbed about what this loss says about me?

Explore where your shame began — was it from your own beliefs, things others said, or a deeper fear?

What are the unspoken messages I've absorbed about what this loss says about me?

_____

_____

_____

_____

_____

_____

_____

_____

_____

_____

_____

_____

_____

_____

_____

_____

If my shame had a voice, what would it say? What is it trying to protect me from?

Begin to hear shame as a part, not a truth. What is its deeper fear or intention?

If my shame had a voice, what would it say? What is it trying to protect me from?

What does my body carry in this grief — blame, anger, numbness, betrayal?

Reflect honestly on how you feel toward your body since the loss, and what it needs from you now.

What does my body carry in this grief — blame, anger, numbness, betrayal?

Who (or what) would I be if shame didn't define this experience?

Explore your identity beyond the loss. Who are you beneath the shadow?

Who (or what) would I be if shame didn't define this experience?

What kind of compassion do I wish someone else had shown me — and can I offer it to myself now?

Gently reflect on how you long to be held, and how you might begin to hold yourself.

What kind of compassion do I wish someone else had shown me —
and can I offer it to myself now?

COOL & RESET

Our nervous system reacts to temperature in ways that can quickly shift arousal. Cool sensations on the face or neck signal the body that danger is passing, helping to calm adrenaline and stress. Spending just a minute noticing the change gives your mind a break from racing thoughts and brings your body into a calmer state — a small but powerful way to regain presence and control.

Find a safe source of cool — a cold pack, splash of water, or even holding something cool in your hands.

Bring it gently to your face or neck. Focus on the sensation for about 60 seconds.

Notice the temperature, the pressure, the way your skin responds, and let your breathing follow the rhythm of the sensation.

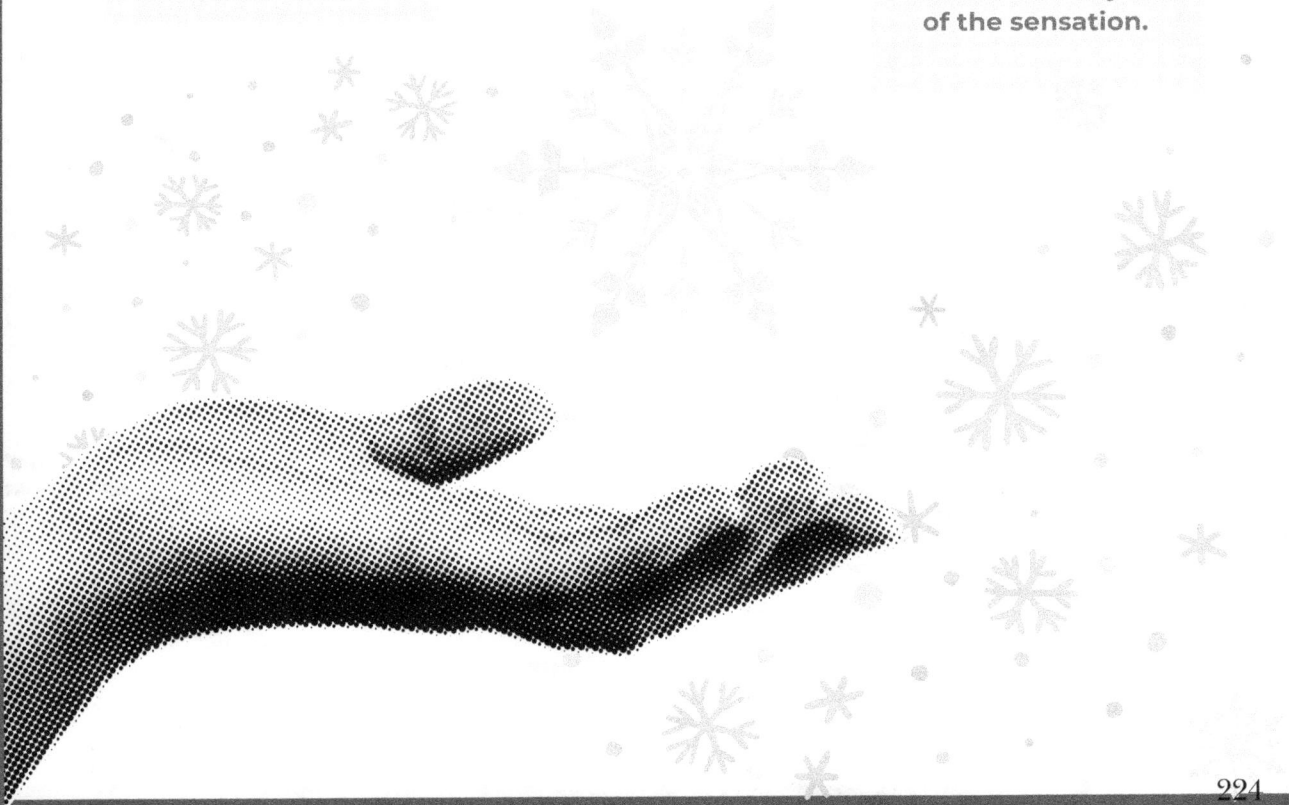

GROUNDING ROOTS

When tension, anxiety, or overwhelm hits, our nervous system often leaves us feeling scattered or unanchored. This simple visualization reconnects your mind with your body and the ground beneath you. Imagining roots growing from your feet into the earth gives a sense of stability and support, while the act of exhaling and sending tension down those roots encourages the body to release held stress. Even a few moments can make your body feel heavier in a good way, steadier, and calmer.

1 Stand or sit with feet flat on the floor.

2 Take a slow breath and imagine roots growing from the soles of your feet deep into the earth.

3 On each exhale, picture tension, tightness, or overwhelm traveling down those roots into the ground.

4 Repeat for 1–3 minutes, noticing the sense of weight and calm building in your body.

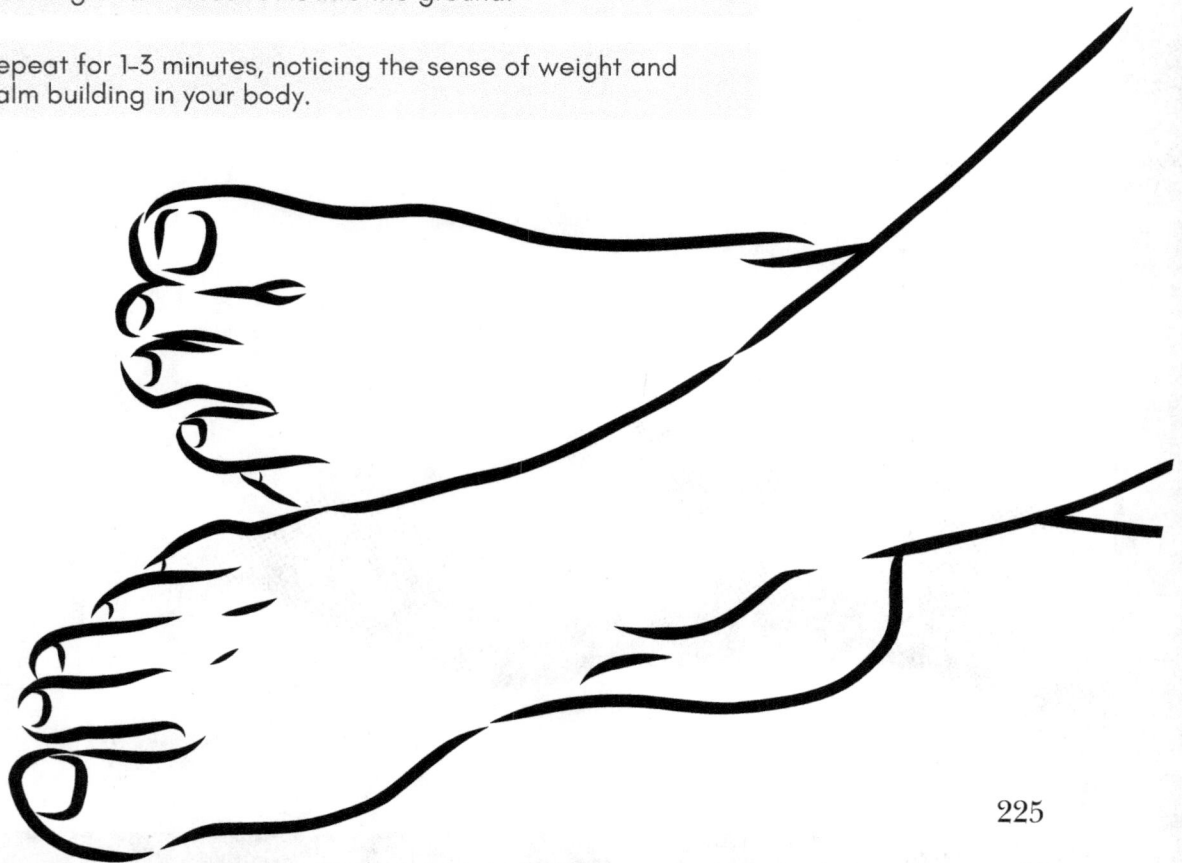

BLUE HUNT

When your mind is spinning, even a few seconds of focused observation can break the loop. Naming five blue objects around you draws attention away from anxious or ruminating thoughts and anchors you in the present. It's a simple, practical way to tell your nervous system: pause, notice, be here. Over time, these micro-moments of awareness strengthen your ability to interrupt spirals before they escalate.

1 Look around your environment and quickly spot five items that are blue.

2 Say each one out loud or in your head: "blue mug, blue notebook, blue pen..."

3 Notice the texture, shape, or location as you identify each item.

4 Pause for a slow breath and notice any subtle shift in tension or racing thoughts.

SECTION ELEVEN

Letting Go Doesn't Mean Forgetting

Somewhere along the way, we're told that healing means "letting go." But when it comes to miscarriage — to a pregnancy that carried your love, your dreams, your future — what does that even mean? How do you "let go" of a baby you never got to hold, a bond that was real even if invisible to others?

This section isn't about moving on. It's about moving with. It's about making space for grief and memory, pain and love. It's about reclaiming the right to hold this part of your story however you need — whether that's quietly, publicly, symbolically, or spiritually. You are the keeper of this love, and no one gets to define what remembrance or healing should look like for you.

Let's explore how to carry your connection forward in a way that honors the love without staying trapped in the ache. Because letting go of pain is not the same as letting go of love.

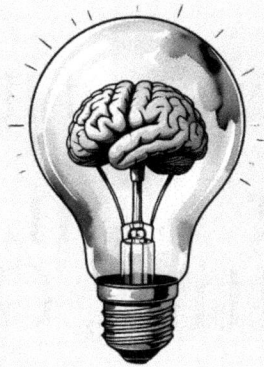

Making Sense Of It
Moving With, Not Letting Go

Much of our culture equates healing with "closure" or "moving on," as if grief is a box to be unpacked and then neatly stored away. Miscarriage challenges that narrative profoundly. The loss is invisible, the attachment real, and the memories — even if only imagined or anticipated — feel tangible. Psychologically, the idea of "letting go" can trigger fear: Does letting go mean forgetting? Does it mean betraying my baby? The mind and heart often resist this, because grief and love are intertwined, and love is not something you can release on command.

Attachment theory offers insight here. Even in very early pregnancies, humans form emotional and physiological bonds. The brain and body anticipate the presence of a child, releasing oxytocin and shaping maternal or parental identity. When loss occurs, these attachment pathways are disrupted, creating profound longing and a sense of incompleteness. This is not a failure or flaw; it is the natural outcome of a deep emotional connection that was developing and real.

Cognitive neuroscience also shows that grief functions as a learning and integration process. Attempting to force "letting go" prematurely can create internal conflict, amplifying anxiety, intrusive thoughts, and emotional tension. Healing in the aftermath of miscarriage often requires integration, not erasure: the ability to hold the memory, honor the love, and still function in the present. This is why moving with your grief, rather than trying to suppress or discard it, is both adaptive and compassionate.

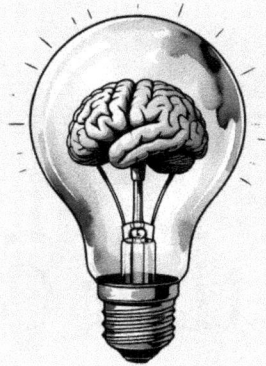

Making Sense Of It

Moving With, Not Letting Go

Socially and culturally, we are rarely taught that grief can coexist with life, hope, and joy. By reclaiming the right to remember, you honor both your baby and your own emotional process. Rituals, symbolic acts, journaling, or quiet reflection can serve as anchors for this ongoing connection. These acts do not perpetuate pain; they provide context, meaning, and continuity — a framework that allows grief to coexist with love, rather than compete with it.

The transformative insight is this: grief and love are not mutually exclusive. You can carry sorrow and tenderness together, holding memory without being consumed by it. By moving with your grief — acknowledging it, witnessing it, giving it space — you cultivate resilience, emotional clarity, and self-trust. You allow your love to remain sacred and alive, while gradually integrating the loss into the story of your life. Healing does not require forgetting. It requires honoring what was real and allowing it to exist alongside what is, in all its complexity.

What does "letting go" mean to me — and do I actually want to?

Explore the pressure to move on. Who told you to? What feels right or wrong about that idea?

What does "letting go" mean to me — and do I actually want to?

What parts of this story do I want to keep with me?

Are there words, sensations, moments, or memories — even brief ones — that feel sacred?

What parts of this story do I want to keep with me?

How do I want to honor this love moving forward?

Reflect on the rituals, symbols, or private ways you might express this love over time.

How do I want to honor this love moving forward?

Is there something I'm afraid I'll lose if I start to feel better?

Gently examine the unconscious fear that healing might equal forgetting or betrayal.

Is there something I'm afraid I'll lose if I start to feel better?

If I could create a quiet space just for this love, what would it look like?

Let your imagination create a symbolic or real "home" for the bond you're still holding.

If I could create a quiet space just for this love, what would it look like?

What does it look like to carry this grief and love together — not in conflict, but in balance?

Describe what an integrated, human way of remembering might look like for you.

What does it look like to carry this grief and love together — not in conflict, but in balance?

TRACING THE TRUTH

MEMORY ANCHOR

When grief feels invisible, creating intentional markers of remembrance can help you honor your baby and your emotional bond. This exercise allows you to externalize memory in a tangible, personal way — something you can revisit whenever you need to reconnect with love without being consumed by pain.

Why it helps:
Creating a physical or symbolic memory anchor externalizes internal grief, making it safer to hold and revisit. It validates the reality of your attachment while giving your nervous system a structured container for emotion.

Choose a medium that feels meaningful: a journal, a small box, a piece of jewelry, or an object like a stone or candle.
Write, draw, or place items that represent your baby, the dreams you had, or the love you feel. This can include dates, thoughts, hopes, or poems.
Take a moment each day or week to sit with this anchor, acknowledging the presence of your grief and love simultaneously.

EMOTION PAUSE & SHIFT

Emotions are powerful signals, but they don't always reflect the full truth of a situation. Sometimes anger, fear, or shame pushes us toward behaviors that make things worse—reacting sharply, withdrawing, or avoiding. Opposite Action gives you a way to step out of automatic emotional reactions and act in a way that aligns with your values and long-term well-being. By pausing, checking if the emotion is justified, and responding intentionally in the opposite direction, you teach your mind and body that you can handle emotions without letting them control you. Over time, this reduces emotional reactivity and strengthens self-trust.

Name the emotion and urge.

Example: Anger → yelling at someone.

Check the facts.

Is the intensity of the emotion justified by what actually happened, or is it amplified by past patterns, assumptions, or stress?

Choose the opposite behavior.

Act in a way that's constructive, compassionate, or gentle.
Example: Use a calm tone, approach the person respectfully, or step away for a mindful pause.

Stay with the emotion.

Continue the opposite behavior until the intensity drops by about half. Notice how your body and mind respond differently.

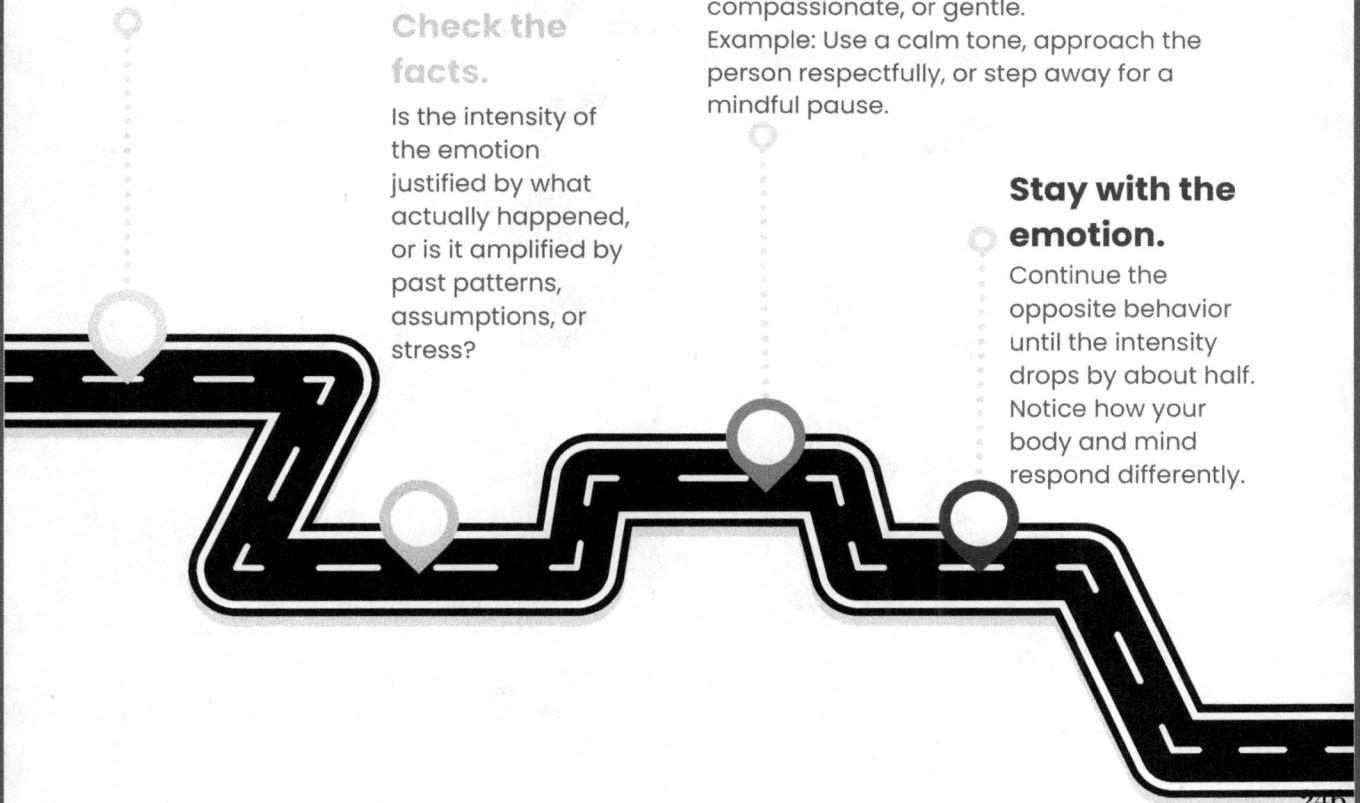

NERVOUS SYSTEM RESET

Sometimes your body gets stuck in high alert—heart racing, muscles tight, mind spiraling—and it's hard to think or respond clearly. TIP Skills target the physiology directly, calming your nervous system so your emotions have space to settle. Using temperature, movement, and breathing strategically helps you interrupt the stress response, release adrenaline, and regain a sense of control. This isn't about ignoring feelings—it's about resetting your body so you can respond thoughtfully instead of reacting out of overwhelm.

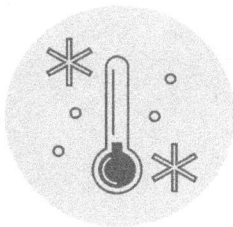

T = TEMPERATURE

Splash cool water on your face or neck, or use a cold pack. This signals your body that it's safe to downshift.

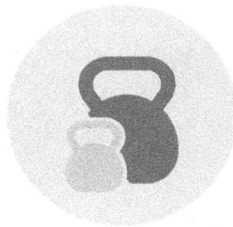

I = INTENSE EXERCISE

Create several posts of the same type at once, schedule them using an app, and upload them so they are available at the right time

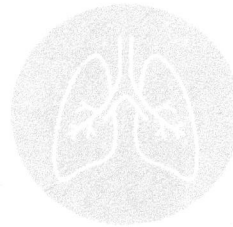

P = PACED BREATHING

You can save time by copying and pasting the CTA into your posts instead of writing it out again every time

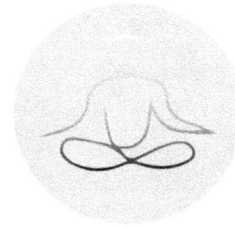

P = PROGRESSIVE MUSCLE RELAXATION

Create some posts with a frame around your branding image. You can reuse the same image after at least 9 posts but change the brand colour for a different look

BONUS SECTION

Redefining the Future – Holding Hope After Loss

When grief first takes over, the future feels like a door that slammed shut. All the images you held — baby showers, tiny clothes, names you whispered in secret — disappear in an instant. It can feel unbearable to imagine "what's next" when what you wanted most has been taken. But grief doesn't mean your life has ended. It means your path is changing, painfully and irrevocably — but not permanently without hope.

This section isn't about tying everything up neatly. It's about honoring the ambiguity, sitting with the unknown, and still allowing a flicker of possibility to remain lit. Whether or not you want to try again, whether or not you feel strong, you are allowed to hope again — not because you've "moved on," but because you're still here.

You get to redefine what the future means for you. You get to heal on your timeline, and carry love with you into whatever comes next.

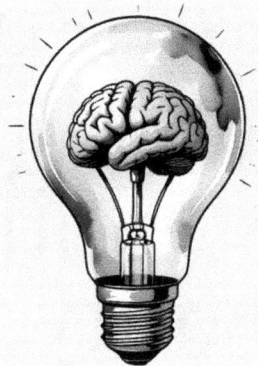

Making Sense Of It

Cultivating Hope Amid Ambiguity

Grief has a way of shrinking time. After miscarriage, the future can feel like a closed door, the path you imagined erased in an instant. Psychologically, this is not just sadness — it's a profound disruption of expectations, identity, and the narrative you held for yourself. Humans are wired to anticipate the future, to imagine continuity, and to invest emotionally in life trajectories. When those expectations collapse, the brain responds with uncertainty, anxiety, and, often, a deep sense of existential disorientation.

Hope, in this context, is not about pretending the loss didn't happen or forcing positivity. It's a subtle, deliberate act of psychological resilience: the ability to hold possibility alongside pain. Research on post-traumatic growth shows that even amid profound grief, individuals can find ways to reimagine life meaningfully. Hope becomes a tool for navigating ambiguity rather than a promise of a predictable outcome. In other words, it allows you to live forward while still honoring backward, holding the memory of your loss alongside the potential for what comes next.

Sociologically, grief after miscarriage often exists in isolation because it is invisible to others. Without public acknowledgment, there is little cultural scaffolding to guide hope or integration. This means hope must often be self-generated, cultivated internally through reflection, ritual, or intentional imagination. Psychologically, these practices strengthen neural pathways that support optimism, agency, and emotional flexibility — all crucial for resilience.

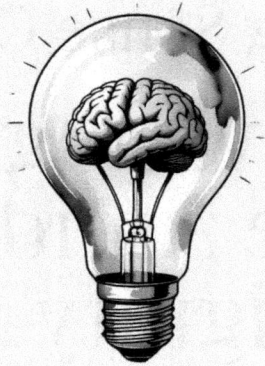

Making Sense Of It

Cultivating Hope Amid Ambiguity

Cognitive-behavioral frameworks also highlight the importance of reconstructing meaning. When the future feels erased, re-framing allows you to create a narrative that is truthful about loss but open to possibility. This can take many forms: redefining family, pursuing new goals, or nurturing aspects of life that were previously peripheral. It is not about replacing what was lost, but about acknowledging the gap while gently exploring what remains possible.

Transformatively, redefining the future is an act of reclaiming agency. You are no longer passively subjected to grief or circumstance; you are an active participant in shaping the meaning, the memory, and the possibilities of your life. Hope is no longer a distant, abstract concept — it is a daily choice to allow yourself to envision a life that holds both the ache of loss and the potential for joy, however it may appear. In this space, grief and hope coexist, guiding you toward a future that honors what was lost while nurturing what is still possible.

What does my future feel like to me right now — and how has that changed?

Explore your current emotional landscape when thinking ahead.
Is it foggy, painful, hopeful, empty, or something else?

What does my future feel like to me right now — and how has that changed?

What future did I imagine before the loss? What feels lost, and what still feels possible?

Begin separating grief from your sense of self — your dreams may be altered, but not destroyed.

What future did I imagine before the loss? What feels lost, and what still feels possible?

Do I feel pressure to make decisions about "trying again"? Where is that pressure coming from?

Gently unpack any external or internal expectations about what you "should" be doing next.

Do I feel pressure to make decisions about "trying again"? Where is that pressure coming from?

What parts of me are scared to hope again — and what do those parts need to feel safer?

Dialogue with the tender, protective voices within that are afraid to be hurt again.

What parts of me are scared to hope again — and what do those parts need to feel safer?

What kind of life do I want to build, even if it looks different than I planned?

Dream forward — not to erase what was lost, but to honor the self who still deserves a full life.

What kind of life do I want to build, even if it looks different than I planned?

TRACING THE TRUTH

LETTER TO YOUR FUTURE SELF

Grief after miscarriage can make the future feel uncertain, even impossible. Writing a letter to your future self allows you to gently imagine what life might hold — not as a demand to "move on," but as a compassionate act of connection and possibility. This exercise helps you hold hope alongside grief, honoring both your past loss and the potential for what's ahead.

Why it helps:
Writing to your future self creates a safe container for hope, allowing you to imagine life beyond loss without pressure or guilt. It validates your grief while encouraging agency and self-compassion. By externalizing your hopes, you strengthen neural pathways that support optimism and resilience, helping you carry both sorrow and possibility forward.

Begin your letter with a date in the future — for example, "One year from now" or "Five years from today."
Reflect on what you hope for yourself: emotionally, spiritually, and practically. Include small hopes — moments of peace, joy, or courage — as well as larger possibilities.
Acknowledge your grief and the ways you've carried your loss. You might write: "I know this year has been hard, and I honor the love I've carried and the sadness that hasn't left me. I hope you are still carrying that love with gentleness."
Close with a message of compassion and encouragement.

TRACING THE TRUTH

LETTER TO YOUR FUTURE SELF

TRACING THE TRUTH

LETTER TO YOUR FUTURE SELF

TRACING THE TRUTH

LETTER TO YOUR FUTURE SELF

TRACING THE TRUTH

LETTER TO YOUR FUTURE SELF

SEEING THE BIGGER PICTURE

When someone's behavior triggers you—or when you catch yourself blaming yourself—your mind often jumps to the harshest story: "It's all my fault," or "They're deliberately hurting me." Compassionate Reattribution helps you pause and look at the situation more realistically. By considering context, other explanations, and human limits, you can soften blame, see things more fairly, and plan a small step to repair or respond thoughtfully. It doesn't excuse harmful behavior, but it frees your mind from spinning in harsh judgments.

Identify the blamey thought.
Example: "I shouldn't have said that—now they're upset."

Consider other explanations.
Context: maybe they had a rough day.
Skills: maybe they struggle to communicate.
Nervous system: stress can make anyone react sharply.

Choose a fair attribution.
Example: "They were stressed, not necessarily upset at me personally."

Pick one small repair step (if needed).
Example: check in calmly, clarify your intent, or take a pause before responding.

BLAMEY THOUGHT	OTHER EXPLANATIONS	FAIR ATTRIBUTION & REPAIR STEP

269

SEEING THE BIGGER PICTURE

BLAMEY THOUGHT	OTHER EXPLANATIONS	FAIR ATTRIBUTION & REPAIR STEP

THE TRIGGER MAP

When you react automatically, it often feels like there's no pause between what happens and how you respond. This exercise helps you slow things down and see the chain of events clearly—what triggered the feeling, the thought that popped up, the urge, and what actually happened. Once you can see it all laid out, you can spot the point where you can intervene next time. That small pause is enough to change the outcome, give yourself more control, and break patterns that have been running on autopilot.

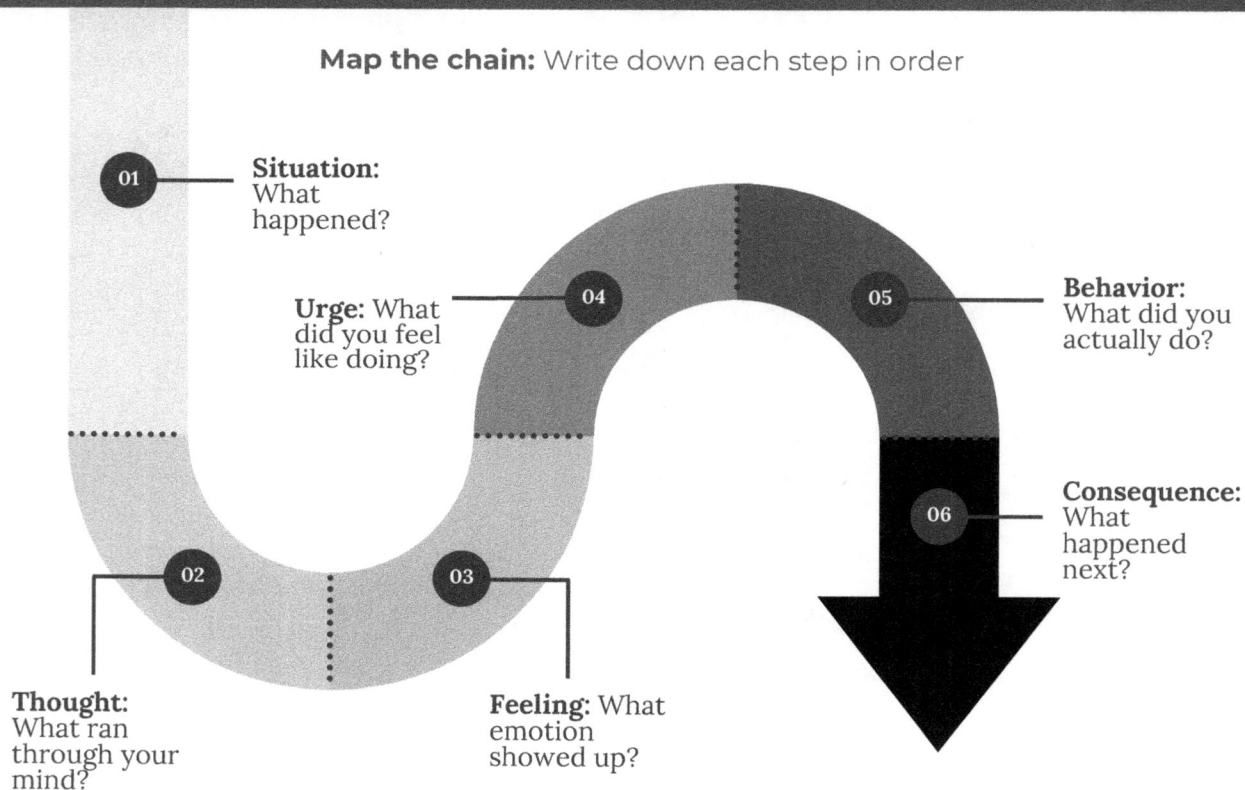

Map the chain: Write down each step in order

01 Situation: What happened?

04 Urge: What did you feel like doing?

05 Behavior: What did you actually do?

06 Consequence: What happened next?

02 Thought: What ran through your mind?

03 Feeling: What emotion showed up?

Circle your change point. Look at the chain and find the first step where you could intervene next time.

Plan one interruption. Pick a tool or skill to use—like a short breathing exercise, a script you can say, or a grounding move—to pause the chain and respond differently.

CLIMBING DOWN

When your mind hits you with a brutal thought—like "I always mess up"—it can feel impossible to jump straight to a positive or kind belief. Your brain just won't buy it. This exercise gives you a middle ground. By writing the harsh thought at the top and gradually stepping down to gentler, more realistic versions, you give yourself space to find a statement that actually feels believable. Even if it's not perfect, that 70% believable thought is enough to lower the intensity and guide you toward calmer choices today.

Write the harsh thought at the top rung. (e.g., "I always mess up.")
Step down slowly. Each rung is a slightly softer, more balanced version of the thought.

"I mess up sometimes, but not always."
"Everyone makes mistakes. Mine don't erase the things I do well."
"I can learn from this and try again."

Pick the rung that feels about 70% true. You don't have to land at the bottom. Just stop where it feels believable.
Act from that rung. Let today's choices come from this steadier, more grounded statement.

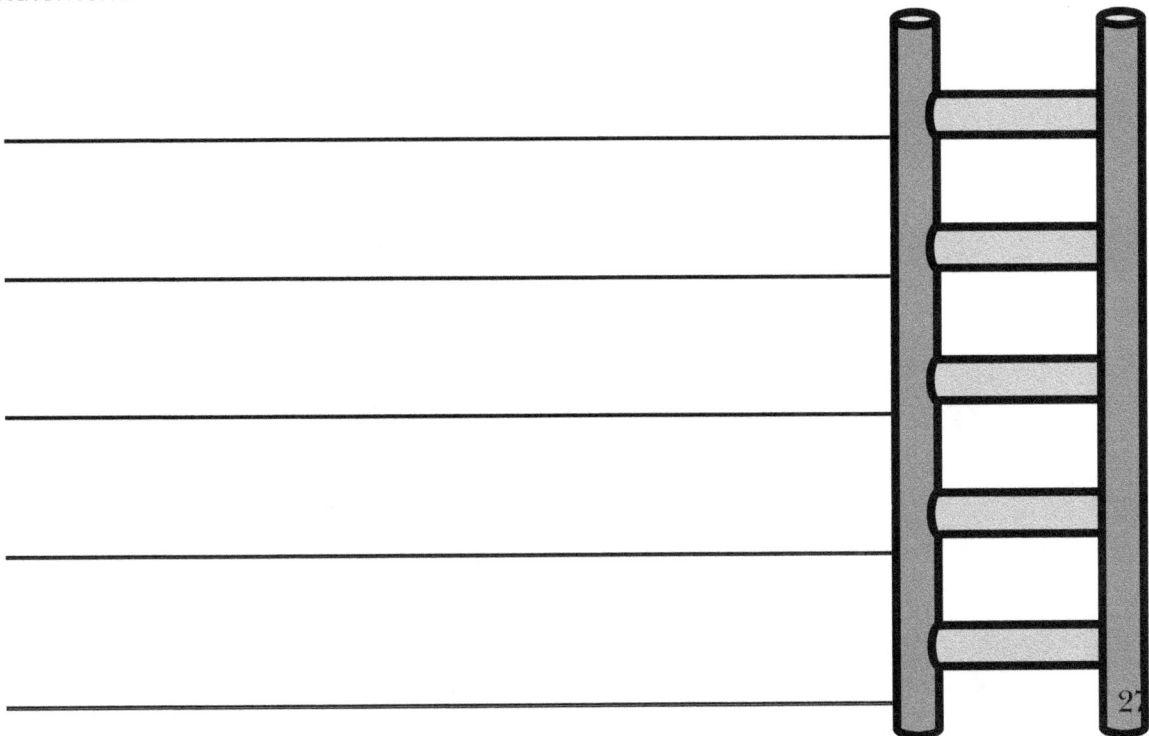

272

ASSESSMENT

You've done the work — now let's see where you're at. Take a moment to rate these statements again with honesty and self-compassion. Notice what's shifted, what still feels raw, and what that means for your next steps.

1-10

1   I feel able to acknowledge and sit with my grief without judgment.

2   I feel compassion for myself when I experience shame, guilt, or self-blame.

3   I feel able to talk about my miscarriage with others in a way that feels safe and supported.

4   I am able to hold my love for the baby I lost while also engaging in my daily life.

5   I feel capable of imagining a future that includes hope, joy, or possibility.

6   I feel I can honor my grief through rituals, memory practices, or reflective exercises.

7   I am able to notice and regulate my emotional and bodily responses when grief arises.

8   I feel empowered to define my healing process on my own terms, without pressure from others.

Mindset & Identity Shift Reflection

Healing changes the way you see yourself. You might notice you're less reactive in certain moments, more confident speaking up, or simply softer with yourself. This page is about spotting those shifts — the ones that show you're not the same person who started this journey.

In what ways do I see myself differently than when I started?

What beliefs about myself or others are shifting?

How has my sense of hope, strength, or trust evolved?

ACTION PLAN

This is your personalized roadmap for continuing growth beyond this workbook. Use this space to clarify which skills you'll keep practicing, how you'll notice early warning signs, and what concrete steps you'll take to support yourself. Remember, transformation happens one intentional step at a time.

Skills I will keep practicing regularly

Early warning signs or triggers I'll watch for:

When I notice these signs, here's what I will do:

ACTION PLAN

This is your personalized roadmap for continuing growth beyond this workbook. Use this space to clarify which skills you'll keep practicing, how you'll notice early warning signs, and what concrete steps you'll take to support yourself. Remember, transformation happens one intentional step at a time.

Ways I can check in with myself to monitor progress (daily, weekly, monthly):

People or supports I will reach out to if I need encouragement or accountability:

One commitment I'm making to myself right now:

RESOURCE LIST

The resources listed here are shared for informational purposes only. While they provide valuable support and tools for mental health, I am not endorsing or guaranteeing the quality, effectiveness, or availability of their services. It's important to explore these options and verify the details directly on their websites to ensure they align with your personal needs.

National Alliance on Mental Illness

www.nami.org

Offers free mental health education, peer support, and a 24/7 helpline.

Insight Timer

www.insighttimer.com

A free meditation app with thousands of guided meditations, music, and talks on mental well-being

Parenting for Mental Health

www.parentingformentalhealth.com

Offers resources, training, and advice on how parents can support their child's mental health, including guides and printable resources

Crisis Text Line

www.crisistextline.org

Offers free, 24/7 text-based support for mental health crises

7 Cups

www.7cups.com

Offers free, anonymous online chat with trained volunteers, as well as paid therapy with licensed professionals.

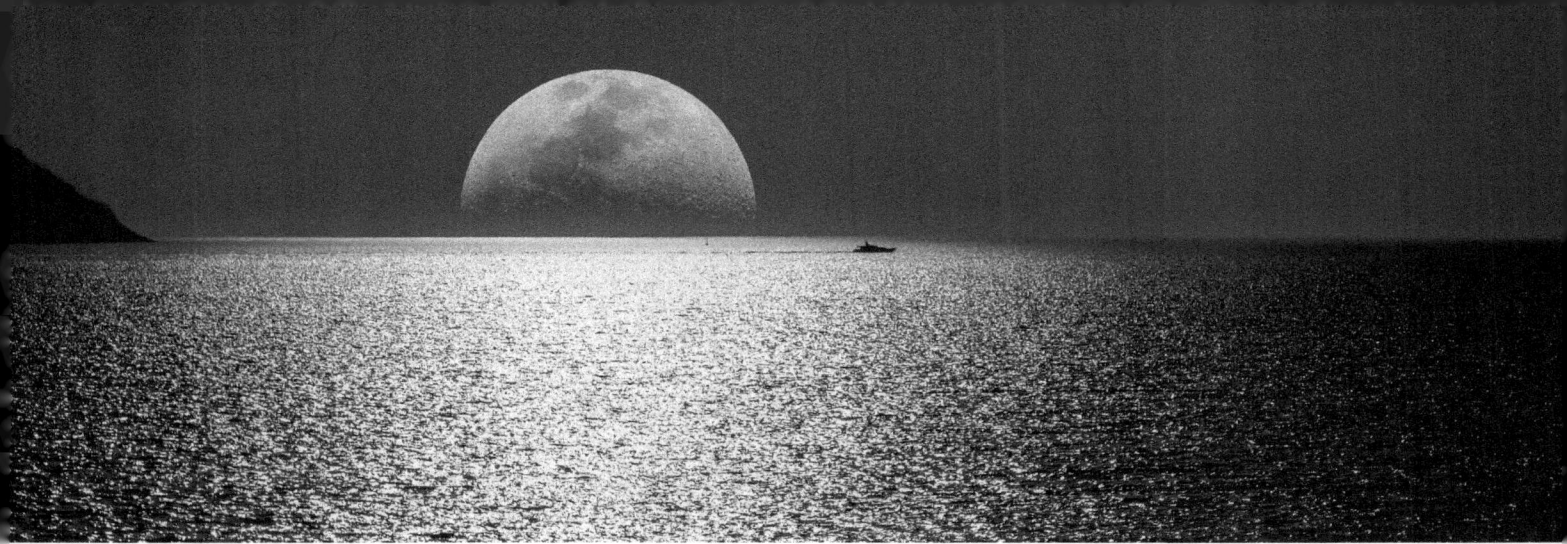

Miscarriage grief doesn't follow clean lines. It doesn't care about timing, logic, or how uncomfortable it makes other people feel. It hits you in quiet moments, unexpected triggers, and the empty spaces where something was starting to grow. You might still feel angry. Or numb. Or deeply sad in a way you can't explain to anyone — not even yourself. Maybe you've tried to talk about it and been met with silence, discomfort, or worse — dismissal. Maybe you haven't told anyone at all. That silence can feel louder than the loss itself. This experience might have shaken things you didn't expect — your trust in your body, your sense of identity, your relationship with hope. That kind of rupture doesn't patch itself up overnight. You don't owe anyone a quick recovery. You don't have to turn this into a lesson, a silver lining, or a spiritual transformation. Some things just hurt. This workbook wasn't meant to fix the unfixable. It was meant to give you space to say what needed to be said — even if no one else was listening.

You're allowed to carry this with you, even if it never makes sense.
You're allowed to shut the door on people who didn't show up.
You're allowed to feel whatever you feel, for as long as it lasts.

This kind of grief can change you — but don't let it consume you. Let the memory live in the way you carry yourself, in the love you offer others, and in the tenderness you learn to give yourself.

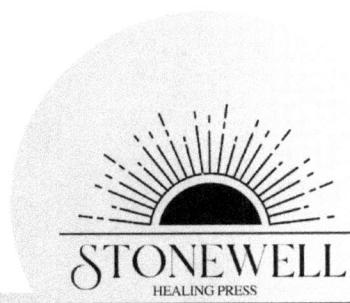

M. Tourangeau
Stonewell Healing Press

STONEWELL
HEALING PRESS

www.ingramcontent.com/pod-product-compliance
Lightning Source LLC
Chambersburg PA
CBHW080131270326
41926CB00021B/4432